BOOTS

BIBS

&

BARBELLS

By Jamie Morrison

ISBN: 0-9844296-6-0

Thank You

To All the inspiring women
out there living with the
strength and courage to
tackle life courageously
without giving up.

Dedication

To those that have loved me in my times of weakness, those that left me when I needed a friend and those that support me through thick and thin. Each of you have given me strength in some way.

**BOOTS
BIBS
BARBELLS**

TABLE
OF
CONTENTS

YOUR
NEW
JOURNEY

If you can push past the pain of your journey you will find yourself achieving more than you ever dreamed.

-JAMIE JAI

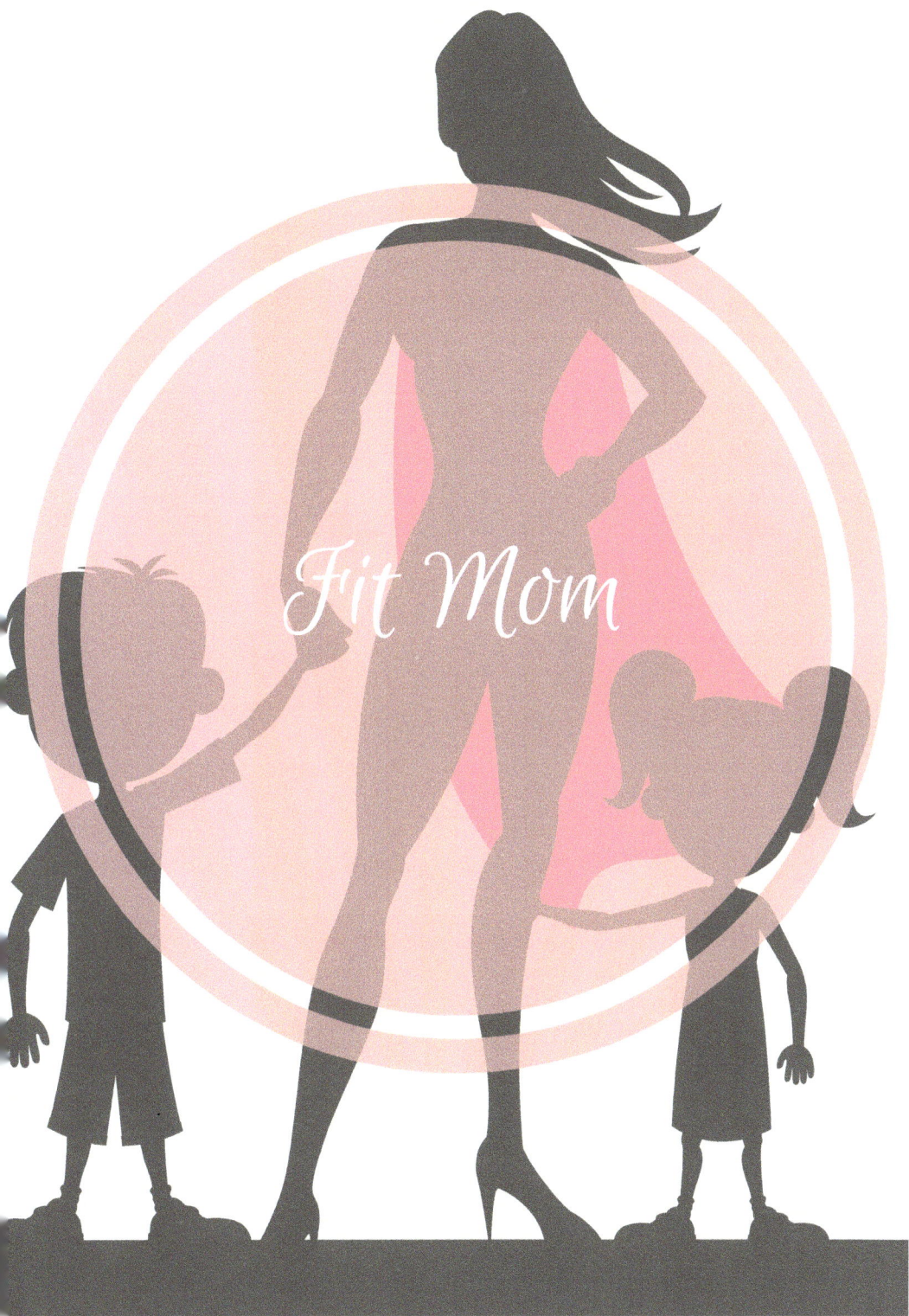

Fit Mom

Have you ever been so overwhelmed with life that you just burst into tears right in front of your Weeples? Yes, Weeples, your children the wee people. Well, I have.

Learning to balance work, fitness, and parenting is a difficult task, and many women sacrifice all to just barely survive with their sanity intact. I'm here to tell you it all can be done. All it takes is a little organization, dedication, and a lot of patience.

This epiphany started when I began my Masters in Physician Assistant Studies. My husband had deployed, my mother-in-law left, moved back to Maryland, and here I was with two very young energetic children; with their gymnastics and swim lessons.
Before becoming the sole parent, I had a lot of time to focus on school and fitness, but now I had to rearrange life. I knew right off the bat that giving up wasn't an option. The only problem was that I had no idea how to get everything on track.

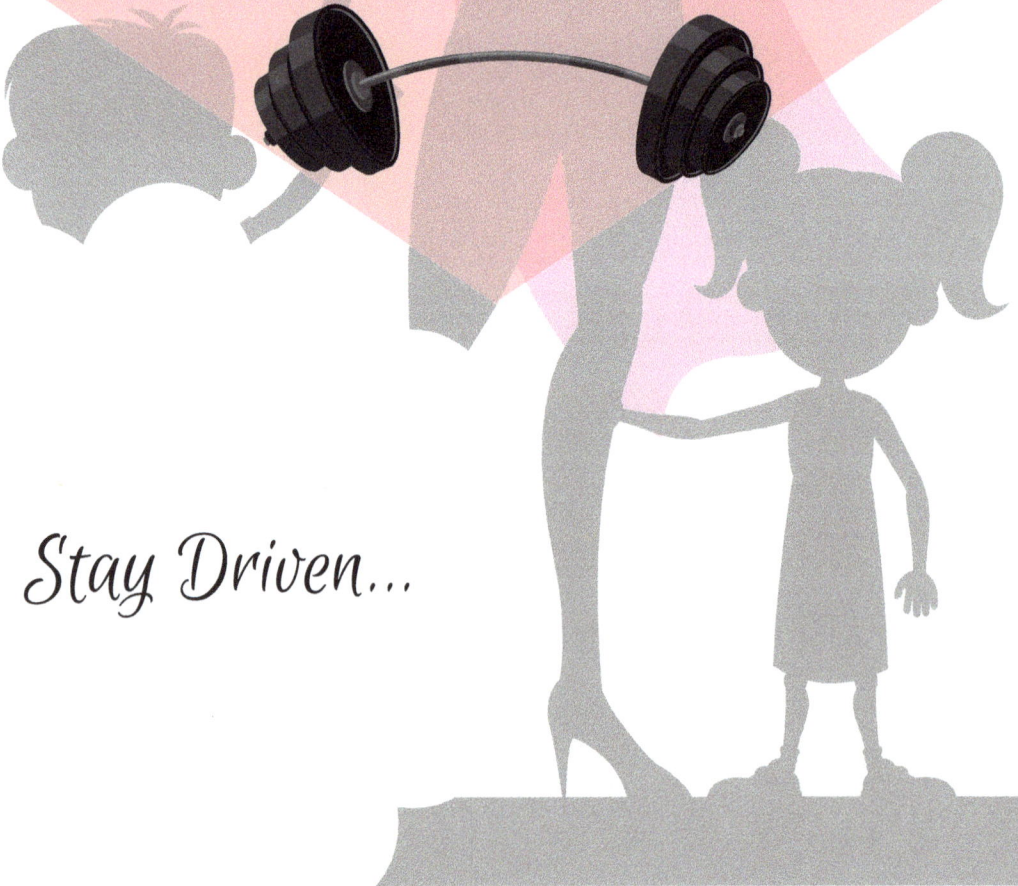

Stay Driven...

One morning, while saying yes and no to the several requests and tattling that the Weeples dished out, I broke down in tears. Yes, guys, I cried like a baby in front of my babies.

At first, they looked at me like, what the heck is her problem (exactly how I look at them during their tantrums). Then they asked what was wrong and I went on to tell them how I had to do so much and how mommy was so overwhelmed.

Do know what they said? "Mommy it's going to be okay." Right out the Weeple's own mouths!

I pulled myself together and said to myself, " Heck yea it's going to be ok." At that moment I put an H on my chest and handled it.

From that point on everything fell perfectly into place. All from just making that simple choice to stay driven, dedicated, and positive. So, if I can, you can too!

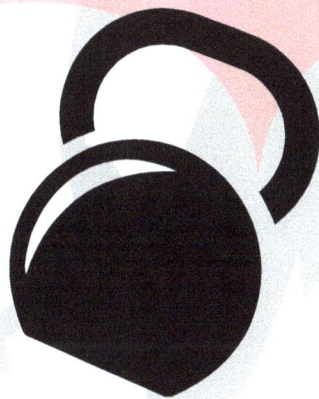

...And Never Give Up!

4

MOVING FORWARD

The journey isn't always easy, but you have to remember why you started and keep dreaming about where you will be afterwards.

-JAMIE JAI

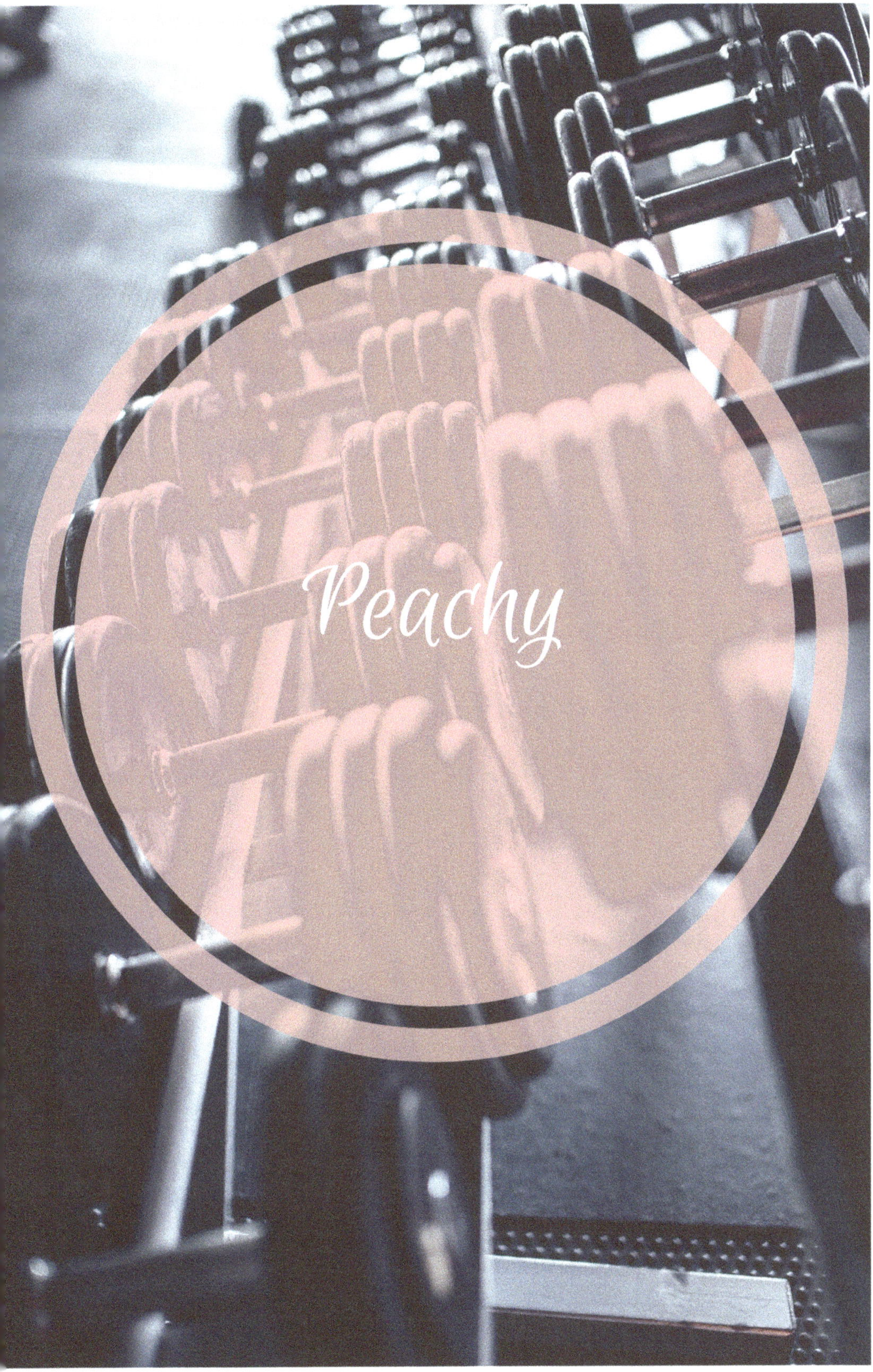

Peachy

Glutes seem to be a treasured body part by all. Women will spend the majority of their gym time growing this muscle group. You have three gluteal muscles, the Gluteus Maximus, Gluteus Medius and Gluteus Minimus. Think of these muscles like a sandwich.

The Gluteus Maximus muscle is responsible for moving your leg towards and away from the midline of the body. Think of the midline as an imaginary line that divides you into two equal halves when standing in the anatomical position. For example, like the bend in a piece of paper after you've folded it. Squats, step-ups, good morning lifts and deadlifts are some great basic exercises to develop your Gluteus Maximus. This muscles lies right over your Gluteus Medius and Minimus.

Your Gluteus Medius muscle sits under and slightly superior to the Maximus. It is responsible for the same movements as the Gluteus Maximus and also stabilizes your hips as well as supports internal and external rotation of your legs. Five exercises you can do to target this muscle would be squats, glute bridges, mountain climbers, lunge split jacks, and plyometrics. Plyometrics are definitely my favorite workout because it involes using your entire body. Meaning, that you are hitting your core and also getting a great cardio workout as well.

When I first started out, I had no gym knowledge, and plyos was just a word. So, below are a few plyos to start you off.

Pyos:

Front Box Jumps
Barbell Squat
Jumps
Burpees
Jumping Jacks
Jumping knee up
down

Gluteus Minimus:

Side leg raises
Hip abductors
Walking side squats

Our smallest glute muscle is the Gluteus Minimus. The Gluteus Minimus is responsible for hip extension, abduction, adduction and is also known for being the primary internal rotator of the hip joint. To give this muscle a good workout you can lie on your side and do bent knee or straight leg side bridges.

Well, what if I'm a stay at home mom and have no time to go to them gym? A gym is not a necessity to be fit and plus this muscle is a small muscle meaning you don't need to use heavy weights to get a good burn. Your own body weight is fine and bands add more challenge to home workouts. You just have to get creative. Below are a few exercises you can do at home and some even at work.

At Home Moms:
Glute Kickbacks
Lateral side leg raises
Air squats

EMBRACE THE CHALLENGE

There will always be an obstacle. Your view of that obstacle determines your outcome. Like hitting your max rep. If you fear the weight and second guess, then you won't get it up. As soon as you own it and get your mind right you reach a new PR. Everything happening in life is the same way. Don't fear reaching your PR in life. In all that you do approach it positively with a beast mentality.

-JAMIE JAI

The Boots

REFLECTION

Have you ever been walking outside and your own shadow catches your eye? Well, today mine did. It wasn't just my own shadow, but also the shadow of my Weeples. I watched as their little feet trotted along with my combat boots. That simple moment symbolized so much for me.

I remember when I signed the dotted line to join the military, and I'm not afraid to admit that education was my main reason. I wasn't lucky enough to have parents to financially support my education desires or guide me through educational choices. Heck, I didn't have them there to guide me through life choices. The choice I made was about survival, and I had plenty of people who doubted me. I'm sure many thought I would end up pregnant as a teenager and never accomplish anything more than just graduating high school.

Looking at this reflection, I now see what was unseen at the time I signed my four year military contract and raised my right hand. I went from walking into basic training with not even a bank account to now a college graduate. All done while serving with two deployments.

NO! It was not fun waking up to the sounds of rockets while deployed. One deployment I remember lying half asleep on the floor of my trailer with my flak vest over me thinking if I got hit, I'd still probably die anyway.

What I can say about all my years in this uniform is it has made me appreciate the little things in life. I pay closer attention to details and remain vigilant. Family takes on a whole new meaning when you don't know the next time you have to take that long flight, with the possibility of never coming home. On the bright side, I've traveled and most off all I have gotten my education. I've made bonds that time and distance cannot break. Both good and bad are all courtesy of the military.

Funny thing is I don't regret it. Knowing that I am providing my kids with a life I never had is my driving force. Raising my right hand allowed me to travel this path of life. So I look at this picture and I wonder how much further these boots can go and will those tiny feet next to them walk in them one day. Or, will the path I have paved push them beyond that and on to bigger and better things...

REMAIN LOYAL TO YOUR GOALS

Remain loyal to the goals you set long after the mindset you set them in has left you.

-JAMIE JAI

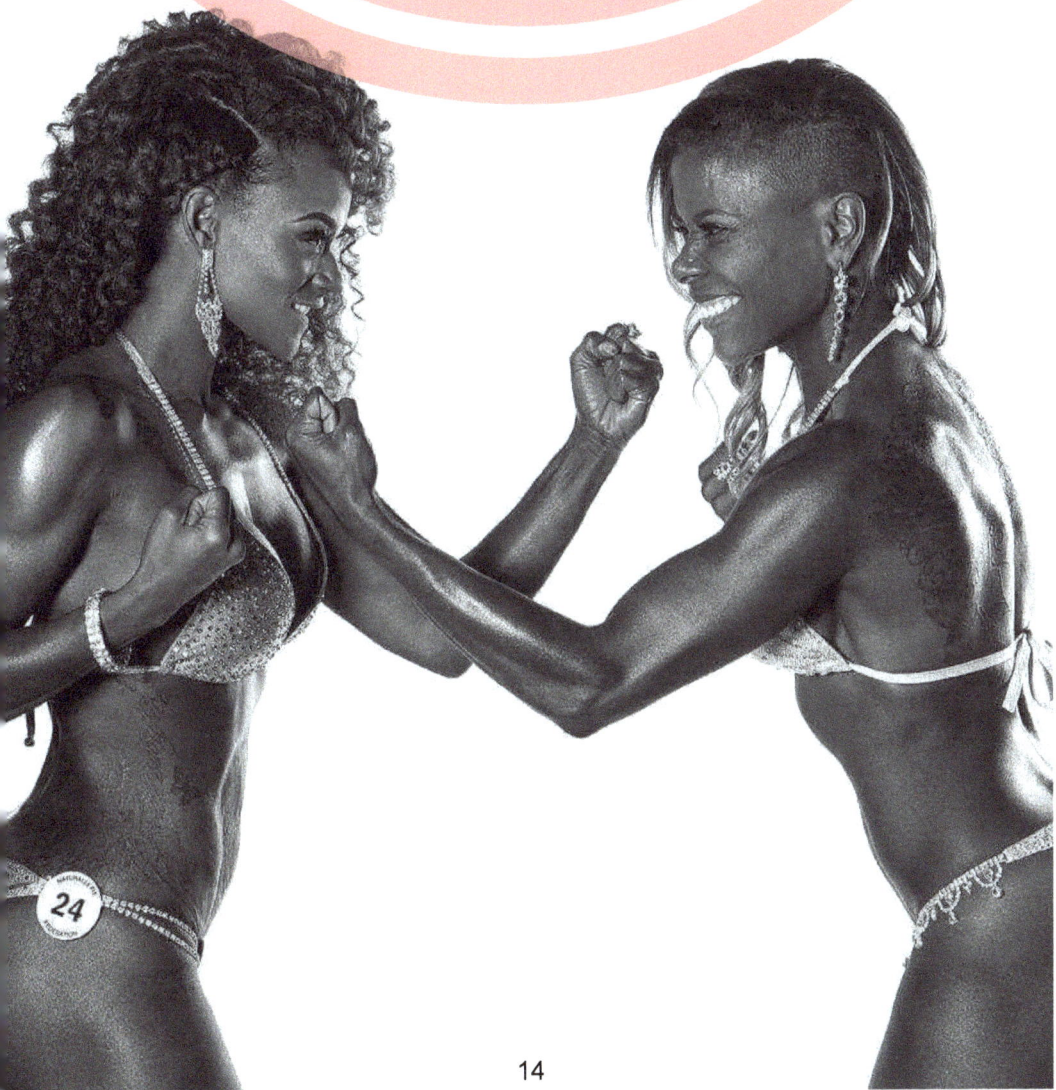

Super Moms

IGNORE THE CHAOS

Chaos comes to distract, and for a moment you feel lost in your thoughts with everything going on around you, but when you quiet the mind, your third eye opens. What you see isn't what you thought it was. Revelations too deep for thought, unrecognizable for the heart, but a perfect epiphany for the soul. Listen to your instincts.

-JAMIE JAI

MIND. BODY. FUEL

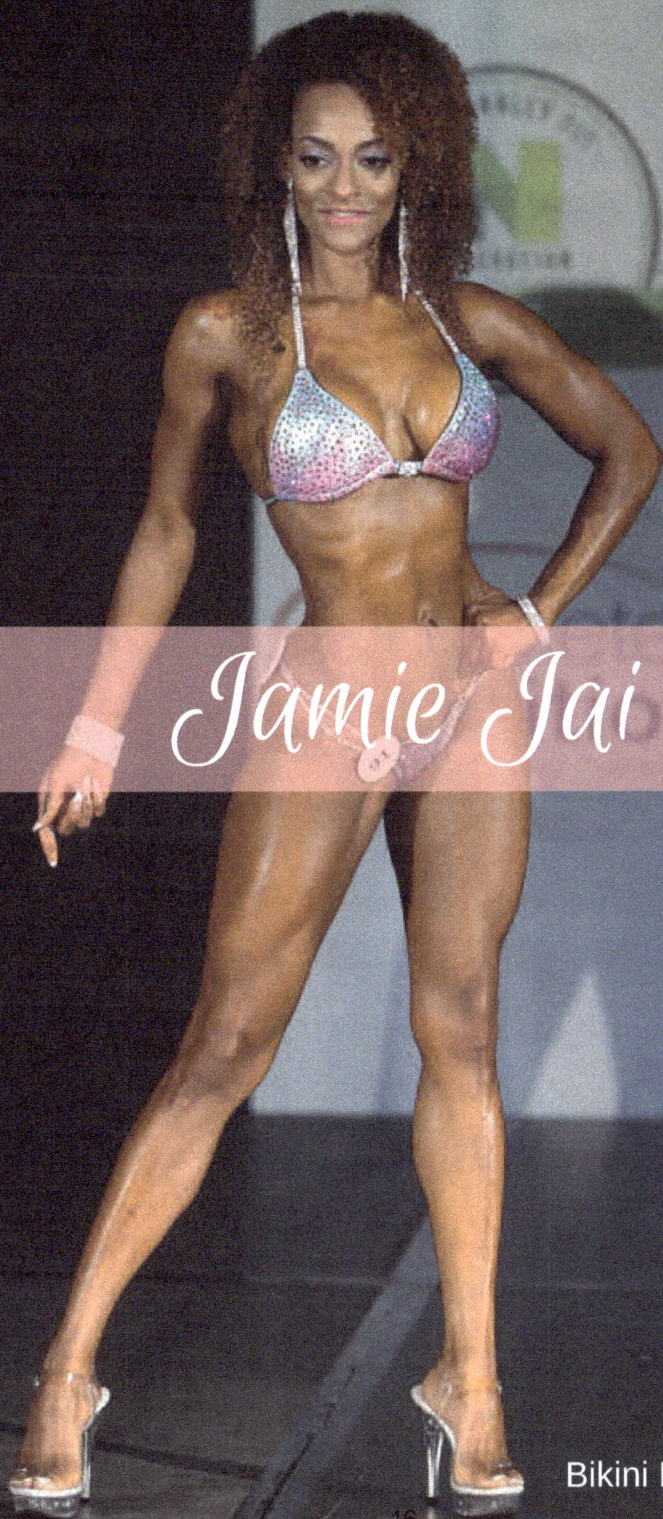

Jamie Jai

Bikini Pro Athlete

16

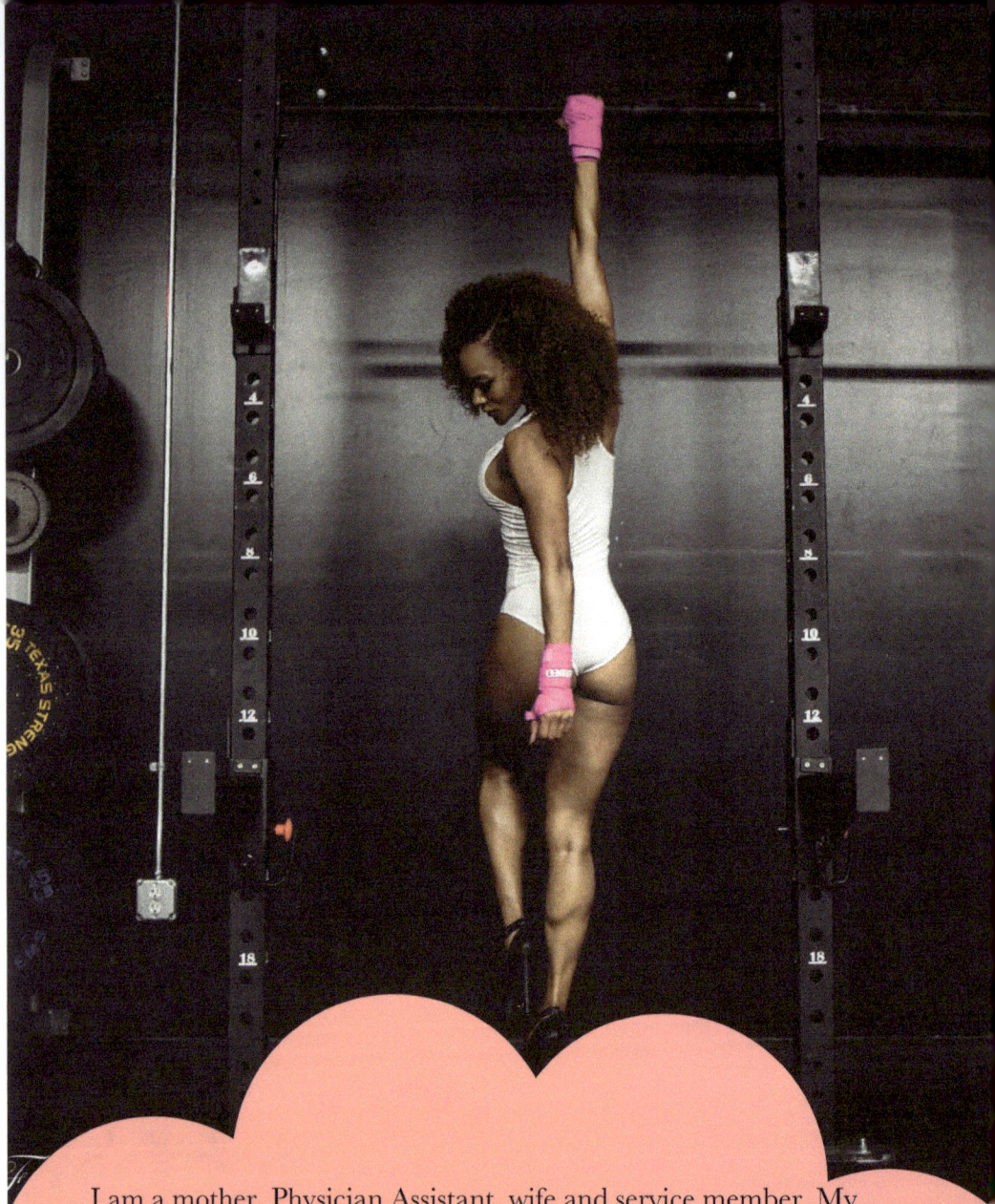

I am a mother, Physician Assistant, wife and service member. My health journey started at the end of 2014 a year after having my second child. I didn't really pay attention to the weight, just enjoyed the food as I gained, but a picture says a thousand words. After looking over pictures from our Vegas trip, I decided it was time to make a change. At one hundred and fifty pounds and sixty-two inches tall, I was the heaviest I had ever been, and I had too much life left in me. Diabetes runs in my family, and I didn't want to continue passing on an unhealthy lifestyle to my children. My family was very athletic in our youth, but as we got older sedentary lifestyles and bad eating habits were our demise.

I had no idea what I was getting myself into, but it turned out to be the best decision I ever made. Not only have I learned to eat better and exercise smarter, but I have also gained some incredible friendships along the way. The best thing is that my children are learning to live a healthier active lifestyle through me. Being a mom, wife, working woman, and student is definitely hard, but I'm here to tell you it is definitely manageable. Today, I can say that I got my Pro Bikini Athlete card and my Bachelors degree a month apart. I placed second place during my pro debut and got my Masters degree within twelve months. I share this to let you all know all things are possible.

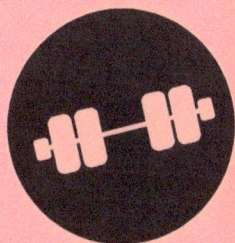

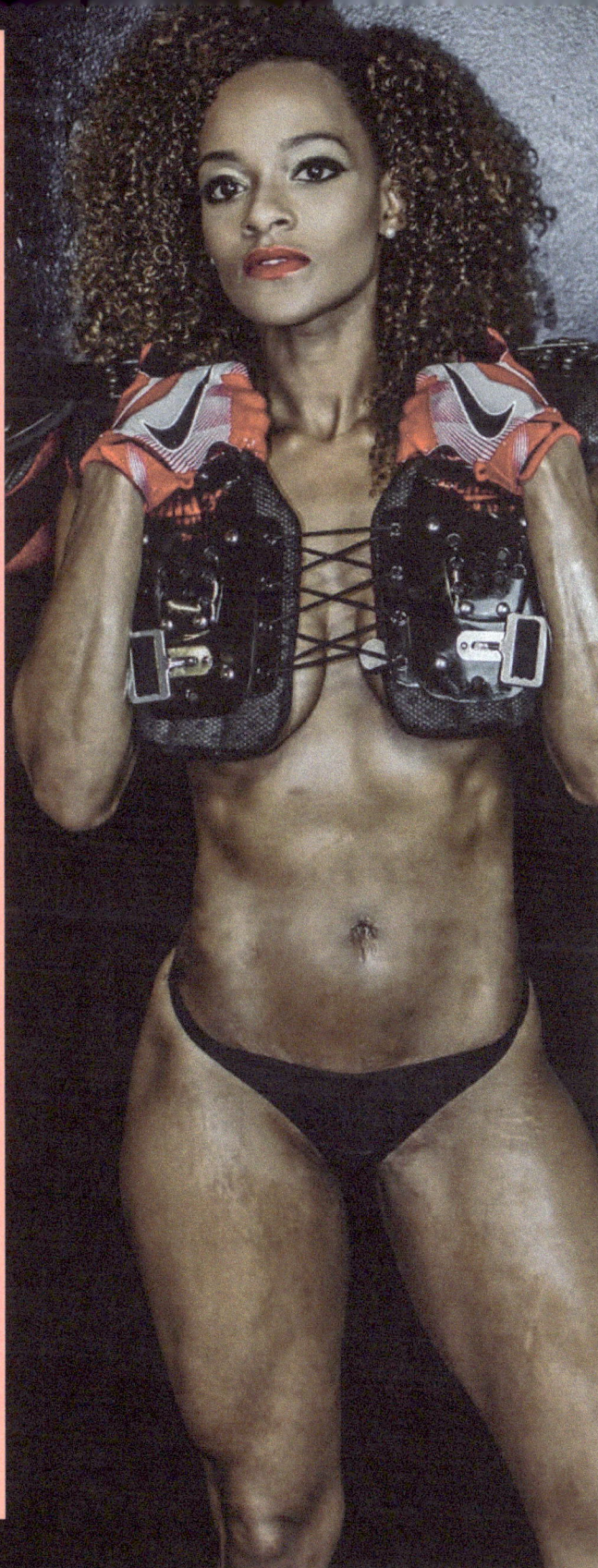

Of course, glutes are by far my favorite muscle group to train. It is one of the most important muscle groups judged in the bikini category.

When I train glutes I always have to incorporate some type of deadlift; mostly the straight leg deadlift. This exercise not only works your glutes but also the hamstrings and back.

First, start out with a comfortable weight to reduce the chance of injury.

Proper form is key when lifting to insure you isolate the target muscles.

You can use a barbell, dumbbells or rack bar.

Keep your back straight as you rise and make sure the movement is from the hips. Squeeze the glute muscles tight as you pull up and repeat.

Favorite

Workout

FAVORITE MEAL

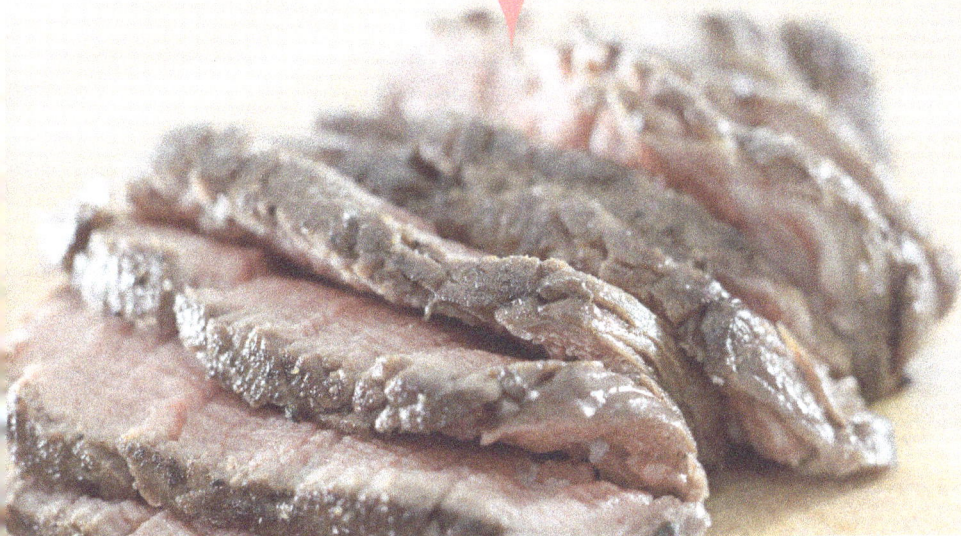

3oz **Thin Sirloin Steak**

4 **Egg Whites**

2 **Slices of Toast**

1 **Tbsp of Almond Butter**

Protein 40.5g | Carbs 26.5g | Fats 10.8g

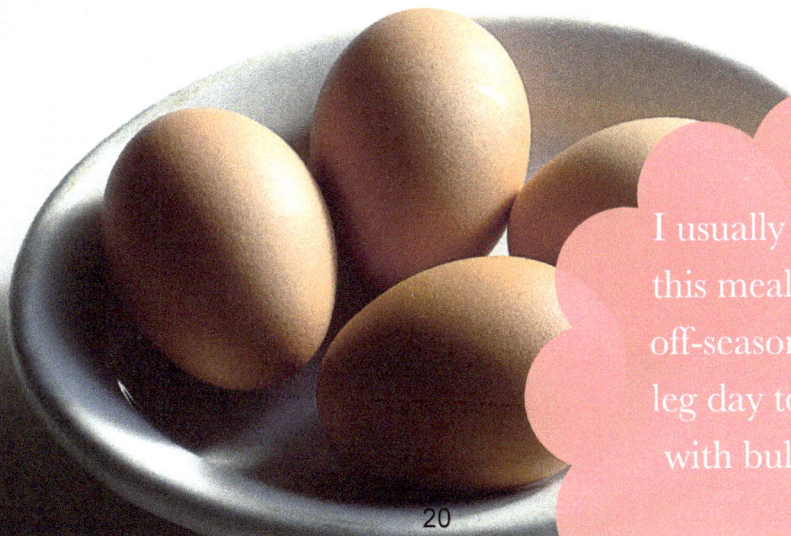

I usually will eat this meal during off-season on a leg day to help with bulking.

COLLECT YOUR WISDOM

Mindset is the name of the game. Don't set your own self up. Everyday is a new day for knowledge. Gain wisdom from the past and apply it to the future. Don't grow old with a young mind. It's a terrible thing to waste. Be wise enough to interrupt the viscous cycle. A new day, a new choice. Knowledge applied. Wisdom gained.

-JAMIE JAI

Health Alert

DIABETES

What is Diabetes?

There are two different types of diabtes; type one and type two.
Type one is diagnosed mostly during childhood and is due to
the bodies inability to produce insulin. Diabetes type two is
more prevalent in adults. Type two diabetes is due to the
bodies growth in resistance to insulin. The cells in our body
need glucose, known as sugar, for energy and insulin is the
hormone that helps glucose get into the cells.

What to look for?

Most people will not have signs or symptoms of diabetes. The
body has a remarkable way of adapting to the elevated glucose
levels. Those that do have signs and symptoms may experience
frequent urination, thirst and blurred vision.

How can I prevent Diabetes?

Regular exercise and a diet low in saturated fats to help
decrease weight has been beneficial as well as limiting
beverages and foods high in sugar. Carbohydrates such as
breads and rice should also be reduced if you have diabetes.
It is important to not only see a health care provider regularly
if you have diabetes but also a nutritionist.

Glucose, or blood sugar, control is very important in the preservation of limbs, life, and eyes sight. Most people only focus on blood sugar level, but this disease can wreak havoc on your entire body.

Of course, poor circulation leads to a decrease in the oxygenation of the organs and limbs. Less than optimal blood flow leads to poor oxygen perfusion of the cells resulting in tissue death. Eventually, vessels began to scar down, skin changes develop, kidneys fail and eye sight can be lost.

Most of the time it starts with a little numbness and tingling at the fingers or toes then works its way more proximal. Intervention is prevention! Obesity, smoking and family history are some big risk factors in the development of diabetes. Smoking along with obesity are two risks you can control. That's right I said, "You". Genetics and lifestyle play a huge factor when assessing one's risk for diabetes, but it is never too early to start practicing healthy life choices. Why wait until your faced with a life or limb decision to make these changes? Regular exercise and diet are going to be the biggest life, or limb, savers.

Not Just About Blood Sugar Level

It's important not to jump into working out without consulting with your doctor. Once you get the green light ease right into it and wear comfy shoes that aren't too snug.

Start with about 10 minutes of training and then work your way up to about 30 minutes. Strength training at least twice a week will definitely help improve your glucose levels.

Remember to be smart about timing your glucose level checks, medication administrations, meals, and training. If you dose yourself with your insulin, do not eat the proper amount of carbs you're scheduled to intake, and then go workout, you're putting yourself at risk of developing hypoglycemia.

Insulin helps your muscles uptake the carbohydrates in your body. Taking your insulin combined with working out uses your bodies readily available carbs leading to a drop in blood sugar. Your brain will signal the body to break into your fat storage to release more carbs, but that takes time. In the meantime, your body needs carbohydrates now and the signs of hypoglycemia will start to set in.

For known diabetics it's important to continuously check your body for any numbness or injuries. If you are hurting then rest. Even if you do everything right, it's always a smart idea to always carry some snacks on you and most of all hydrate.

Be careful not overdue it and watch for the signs that your sugar may have dropped too low. Here are a few signs to look out for:

o Shakiness
o Sweating, chills and clamminess
o Rapid heartbeat
o Feeling lightheaded or dizzy
o Hungry or even nauseous
o Weakness or unconsciousness

Great Foods For Diabetes

BEANS
Great source of protein

GREEN LEAFY VEGGIES
Low in calories and carbs

CITRUS FRUIT
soluble fiber and vitamin C

SWEET POTATOES
Vitamin A and Fiber

BERRIES
packed with antioxidants, vitamins, fiber

TOMATOES
Vitamin C, iron, fiber and Vitamin E

OMEGA FATTY ACIDS

WHOLE GRAINS
magnesium, chromium, omega 3 fatty acid, and folate

NUTS
fiber magnesium and helps reduce hunger

Fat-free Yogurt and Milk
Vitamin D

ROOTS

It can be weird to actually see past the smiles and kind words. Intuition sharp and third eye working. No amount of distance or time makes a bond weak. Bonds that fail were never strong, to begin with. Accept this fact and know that not all things or people are meant to see you all the way through. You are a tree. Those around you are leaves and branches and you know leaves change with the season and branches eventually break. It's the roots. The ones that speak life into you. That pick you up when you are down one, ten, fifty years from now. Those that see you at your worse and love you into your best. A true soldier, friend, and confidant. So, don't cry over branches and leaves. More grow to replace them. It's the roots you need to give your attention to.

-JAMIE JAI

Recipe

Blue Berry Spinach Smoothie Recipe

1 Banana
1 Cup of Blueberries
1 Cup of Almond Milk
2 Cups of Spinach

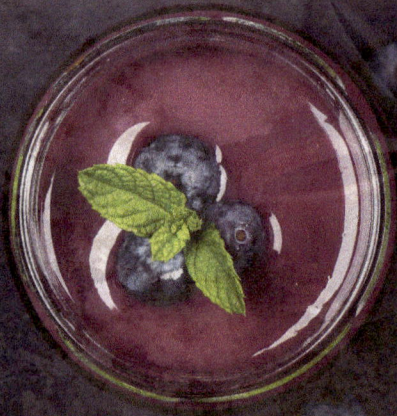

Carbs 26g
protein 3g
fat 2g
Cal: 125

You can freeze the blueberries or buy them frozen to make a cold smoothie. Place in blender and serve.

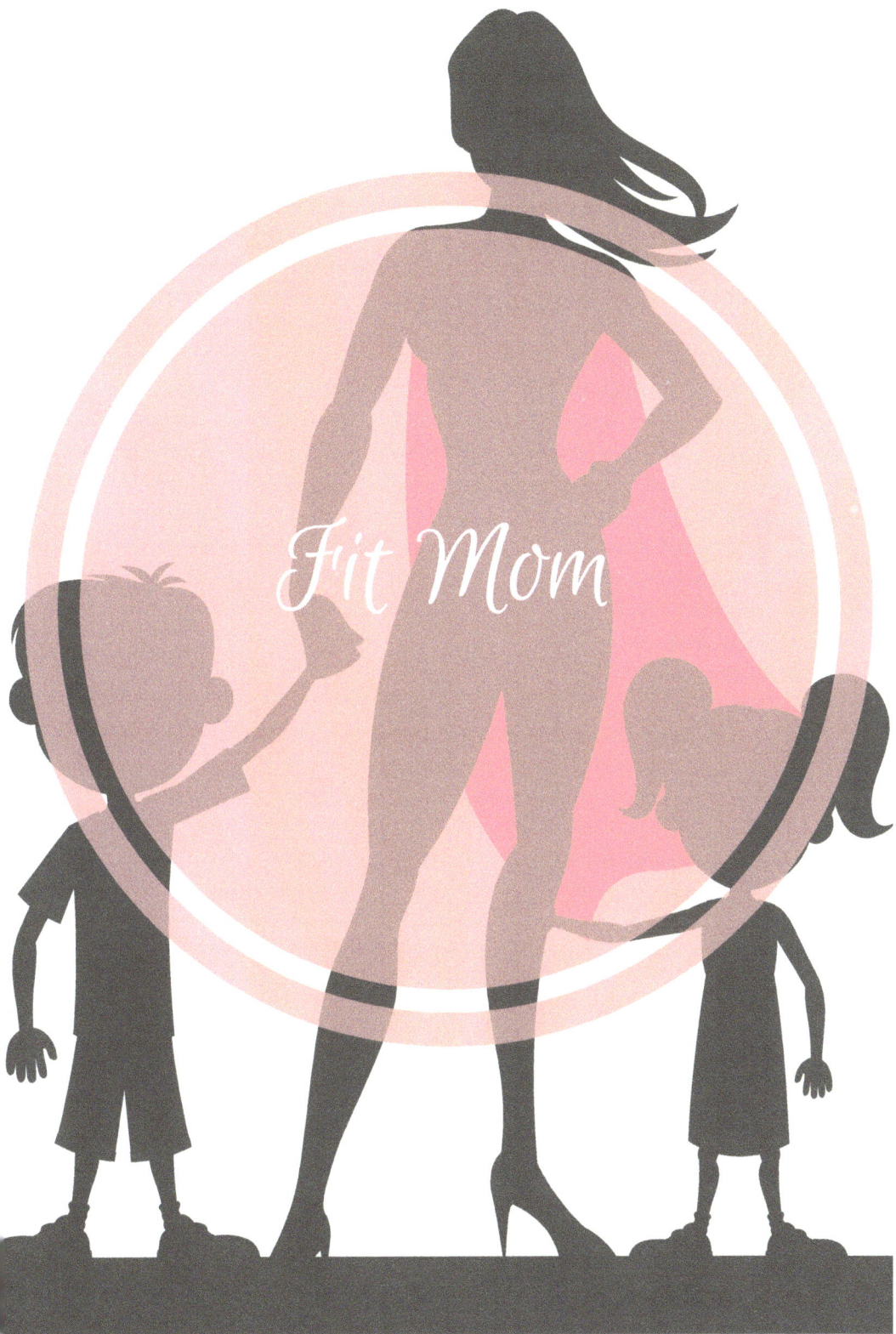

Fit Mom

Preparation is Key

"How do you do it", is the question people ask me the most. I have to be honest with you. It is not easy. April 2016 my Husband got orders to go to Cali and I was left behind in San Antonio to finish school. I was getting my Bachelorette in Science in a sixteen month time period. So, pretty much my life consisted of around the clock studying. Competing and training was my only outlet and we did the best we could flying me between Cali and Texas for family time.

Now I'm completing my Masters in Physician Assistant Studies in twelve months. My husband is deployed which places all tasks on my shoulders. It is hard enough balancing kids, house and work, but on top of that trying to maintain my own hobbies was extremely difficult. I stressed, I cried and felt like I was at my wits end. At one point I felt like I had to give up training, but then "Preparation" was the goal.

Learning to stay ahead is key. You have to prep, prep, prep. Meal prep, Day prep, Night prep, and Gym prep. I knew that if I had a long day ahead of me then the night before I needed to prep all my meals, my clothes, their clothes, their gym meals, and snacks.

Yes, some days I was fatigued after work, but that changed after I got a little pre-workout in while the Weeples ate. That's how you get to the gym, but what about the house and studying?

We all hate doing housework after a long day, but I suggest tackling the most needed task for the night. Wash dishes as you cook. Wipe the table while you clean up dinner. Train yourself to do a little every night before going to bed. I handled studying the same way. Preparation right!

If you set a time for baths, bed, cleaning, and studying you will find balancing it all is not that chaotic. Kids are pretty durable and if you as mom stick to the plan, they will as well. Remember if I can, you can!

Get Into A Routine and Stick To It

REARRANGE YOUR ATMOSPHERE

When you have a positive mindset, people around you with a negative one will pull that positivity from you while dumping in their negative energy. Sometimes you have to know when to let people go. Not out of spite, but out of knowing your own self-worth. If you want a positive outcome, you have to have a positive surrounding. Rearrange your atmosphere. **-JAMIE JAI**

The Wings

Stubborn arm fat can kill your fitness mood, but with determination and persistence you can burn off that jiggle.

Providing the right diet and exercise, your metabolism will start to work for you and not against you, and soon you will be on your way to sculpting the "wings."

Of course, for toning, you should be lifting more for endurance. That means lifting 12-15 reps per set. If you're looking to put on size lift 8-10 reps per set.

Exercises:

o Dumbbell/Barbell Bicep curl
o Cable tricep Press

o Dumbbell Overhead
o Tricep Press
o Triceps Cable/Dumbell Kickbacks

The key is to have fun on your fitness journey and learn what works best for you

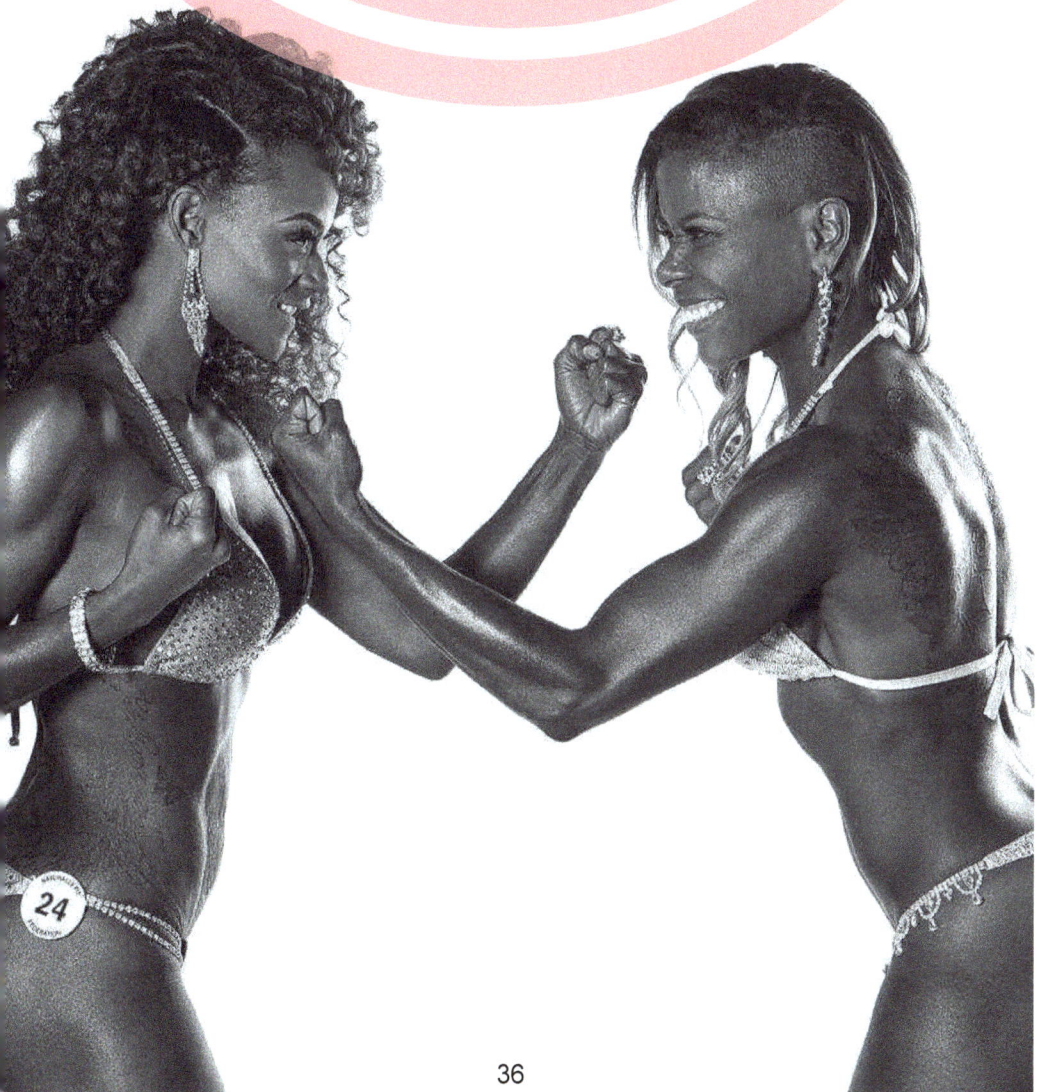

Super Moms

Amanda Miles

Bikini Pro Athlete

Richard G Martinez
PHOTOGRAPHY

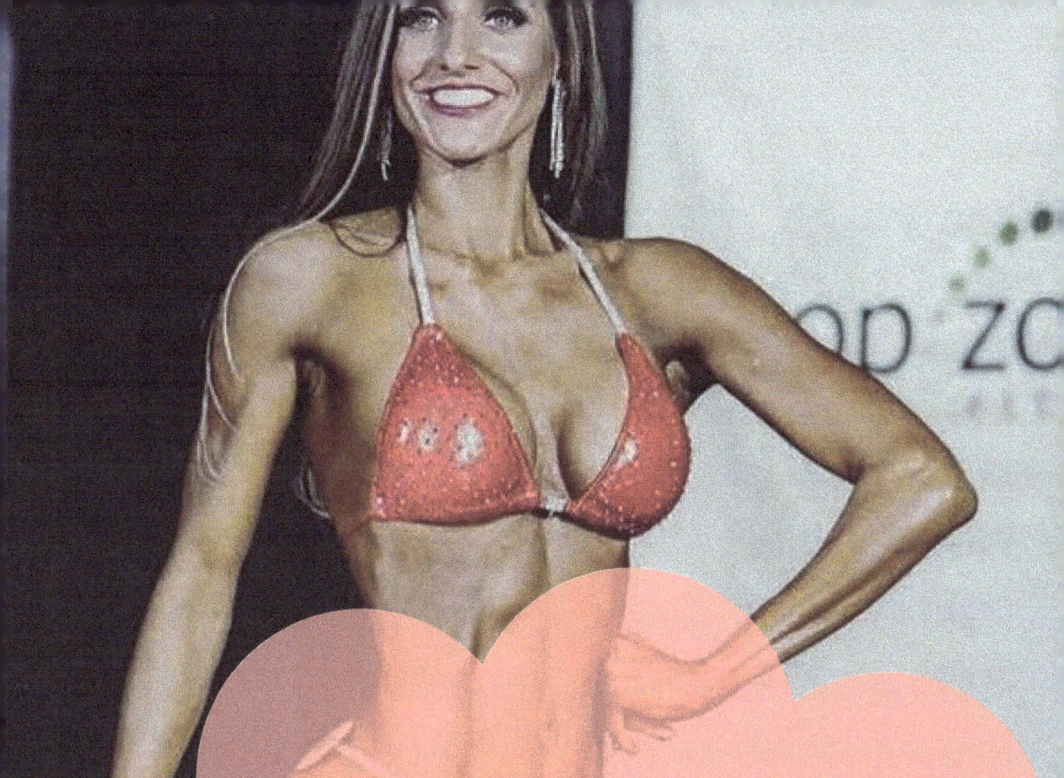

I'm a full-time Mom to two and a baseball coach's wife. I work full-time at USAA as a Senior Banking specialist and am a part-time student at Texas A&M San Antonio working towards my Bachelors in Management with a concentration in Human Resource, and a bikini competitor.

Since I was a military brat, I've been into fitness. I played sports through middle school (track) and some of high school (swim and water-polo team).During college, I would mainly just run. I made sure to continue working out throughout my pregnancies and after. I need the gym in my life, for my sanity.

After I had my son, I started at a new gym and saw a picture of a fifty-five-year-old figure competitor that blew me away. I decided then that I wanted to not just workout but training with a purpose, towards a goal.

Time management is a must with everything that I have on my plate. Since my kids are now in extracurricular activities and I sometimes cannot make it to the gym before the kids' club closes, there are some late nights at the gym and very early mornings.

Most of the time, I have my next two weeks figured out and write down in my calendar. I have high-carb and low-carb days, what muscle group I'm training, what time I'll do cardio (AM or PM), assignments that are due, and all my kids' activities always written down. Honestly, it allows me to have more free time than one would think.

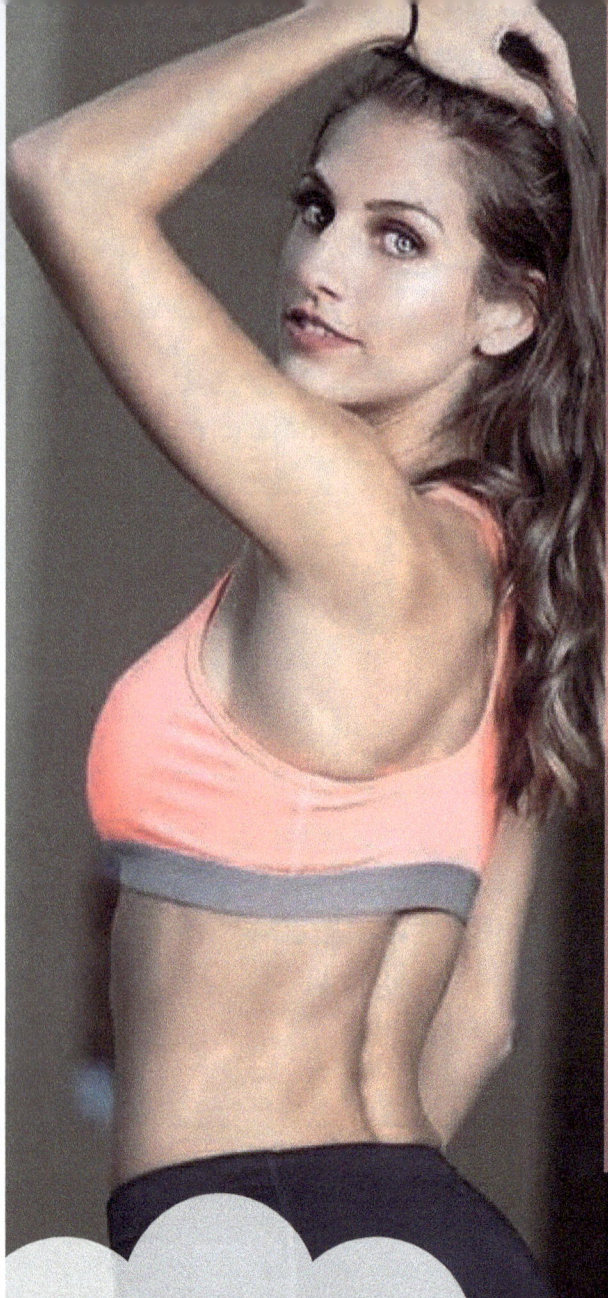

My favorite workout is the dumbbell Bulgarian split squat. The dumbbell Bulgarian split squat is a single-leg strength exercise that targets the quads, glutes, and hamstrings.

To do the Bulgarian split squat, you take one foot back and elevate the top of your foot on a bench (or something that is elevated), and then step out a bit with your other foot and do a single leg squat.

Performing the exercise with dumbbells ensures muscular balance on both sides of the body. I have horrible balance so, not only does it help me strength wise, but it has helped with my balance. Hello, yoga! Well no yoga, yet.

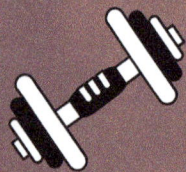

Favorite Workout

FAVORITE MEAL

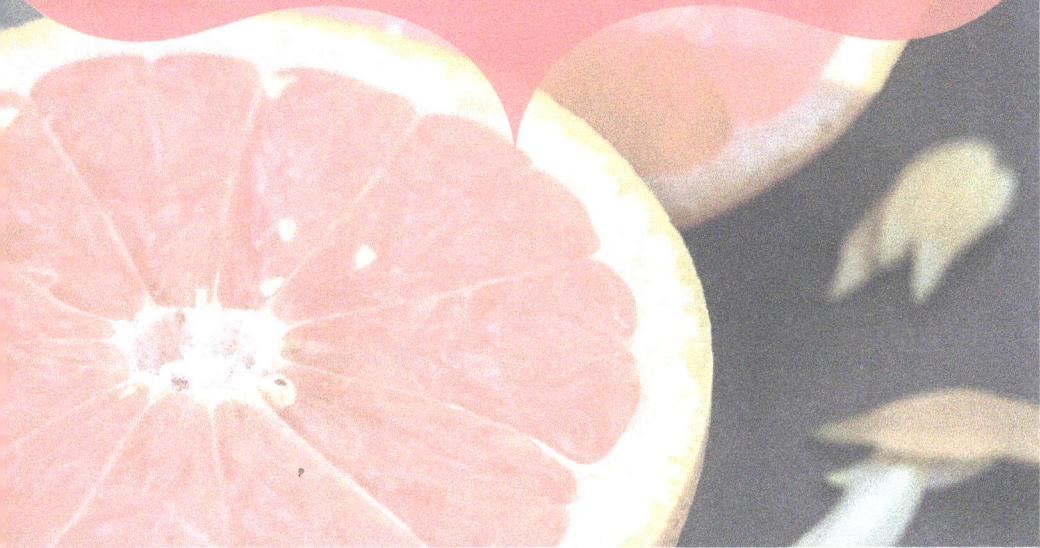

1 Cup Almond Milk
140g Egg Whites
37g Dry Oats
1/2 Small Grapefruit

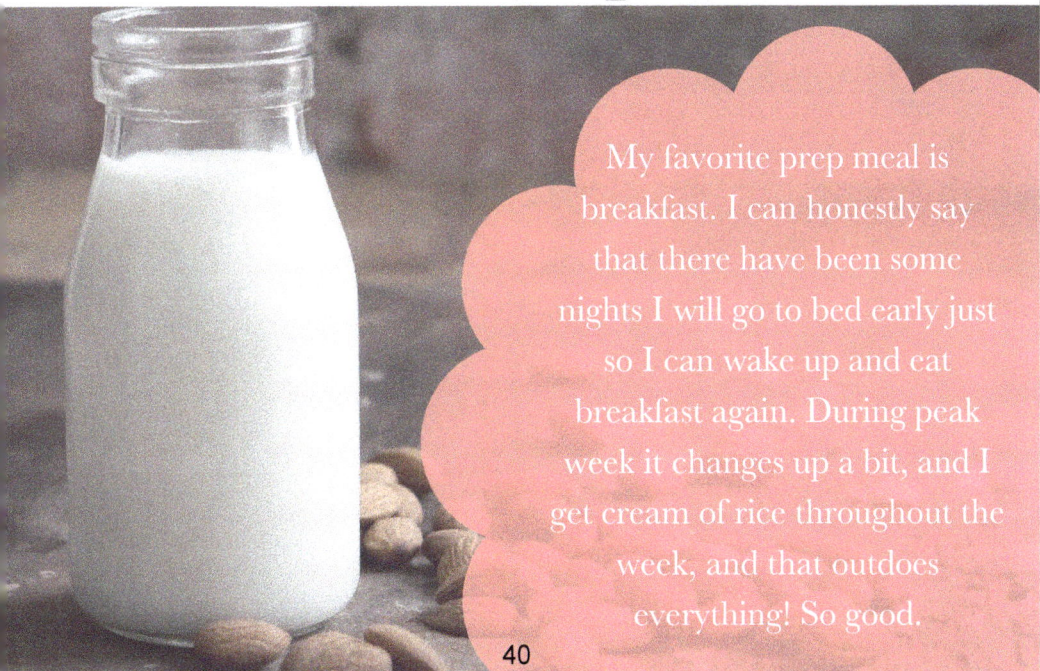

My favorite prep meal is breakfast. I can honestly say that there have been some nights I will go to bed early just so I can wake up and eat breakfast again. During peak week it changes up a bit, and I get cream of rice throughout the week, and that outdoes everything! So good.

SCATTERED PIECES

Not every moment of your journey will you feel like you have it all together. A lot of people put on a happy face, but deep down inside feel like they are barely holding together the small pieces of life. This is a normal feeling. When stepping out of your comfort zone feeling lost, overwhelmed or scattered is normal. It is the beauty of the new; that is, the new you, new life, new dreams, a new path. It's a masterpiece in the making! Nothing great comes easy.

-JAMIE JAI

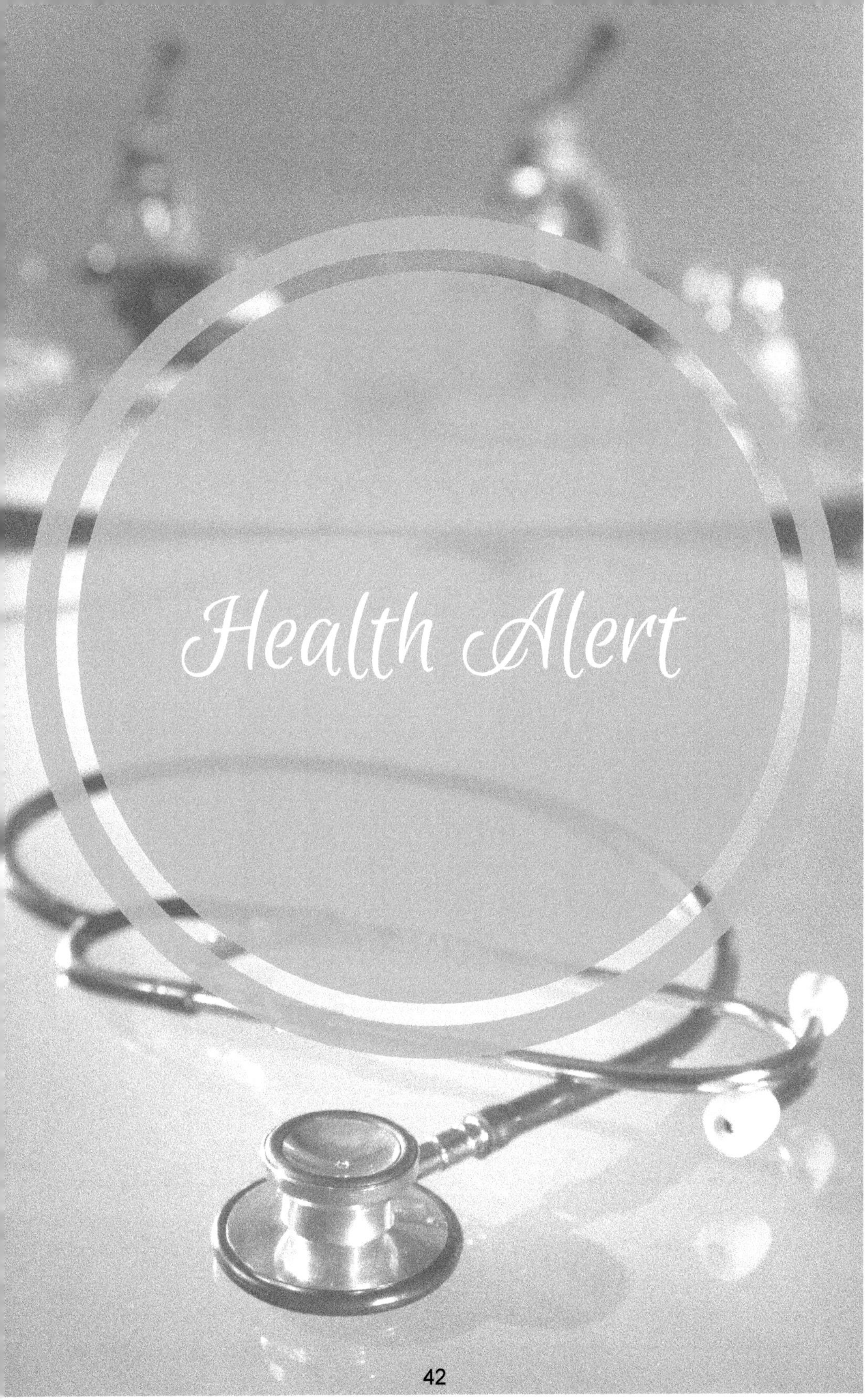

Health Alert

What is high blood pressure?

High blood pressure is also known as Hypertension. It is a condition in which the blood pressure, the force of blood beating against the blood vessels walls, is constantly elevated. I have had several patients come in and call their blood pressure the "Top number" or "bottom number." Well, your systolic blood pressure, the top number, is the pressure exerted on your arteries while your heart is contracting. The diastolic, bottom number, is the pressure in your arteries when your heart is at rest between beats.

How can I lower my blood pressure?

It's not a huge secret that exercise and healthy eating can have positive effects on high blood pressure. Regular exercise can help your high blood pressure fall into a more normotensive to the mild hypertensive range. Exercising regularly can lower your blood pressure (systolic or diastolic) by 10/5mmhg.

Why is blood pressure control important?

When you allow the force of pressure beating against your arteries to increase it will over time damage and weaken the artery wall. The damage can lead to aneurysms, stroke or heart attack.

HYPERTENSION

KNOWING YOUR
Risk Factors

What are my risks factors?
One of the biggest risk factors for many diseases is smoking.
Excess salt intake, family history, excess body weight and alcohol
can are also common risk factors for the development of high
blood pressure. All, but family history, are risk factors you can
control.

Talk to your provider about smoking cessation programs and
start to monitor your daily salt intake. Drink alcohol responsibly
and if you need help you can reach out to your health care
provider for that as well. Most of all! Established a workout
routine and be consistent.

Should I exercise?
Yes! Some people think that you have to jump out there and lift a
gang of weights and run a few miles to improve blood pressure,
but that isn't true. The most effective exercises for high blood
pressure are isotonic exercises such as walking and running. A
mild brisk walk 30-60 minutes a day is better than doing isometric
(weight training) exercise. With uncontrolled high blood pressure
isometric exercises can increase blood pressure. Be aware of your
body when working out and always remember to get approval
from your doctor before starting a new exercise regimen.

MASTER OR PREY

Many will come to dim your light, but once you peel back the loose layers of skin, you see the teeth of a wolf. Fear not, because now with that knowledge you become even more powerful. What was meant to break you just lights your path to self-actualization. Become the master and not the prey. True growth... Real power... No limits

-JAMIE JAI

Out Of

Time

Whether you're a single mom, married or just a working woman days can get hectic and you find your self out of time. Lack of time is the most common reason we skip out on a workout. When you break down the math you in fact have plenty of time. It's just about how you manage your time.

There are twenty four hours in one day. We sleep any were from five to eight of those hours, work about ten of them and that leaves you with six hours to work with. Doesn't sound like much, but it's a misuse of time.

I have found that teaching my self to slowly wake up a little earlier each day helps me use that extra time to either be better prepared for the day or actually workout. Having things ready for the day cuts out the time spent gathering things in a rush. When I decide to do my workout in the morning I go to the gym or workout at home. I recommend keeping some light weights and a set of resistance bands at home. Also, investing in a stationary bike or treadmill is a lifesaver. You can also do isometric exercises using your own body weight or your light weights. No action, because of time, means no success.

Getting It

In

Isometric Exercises:

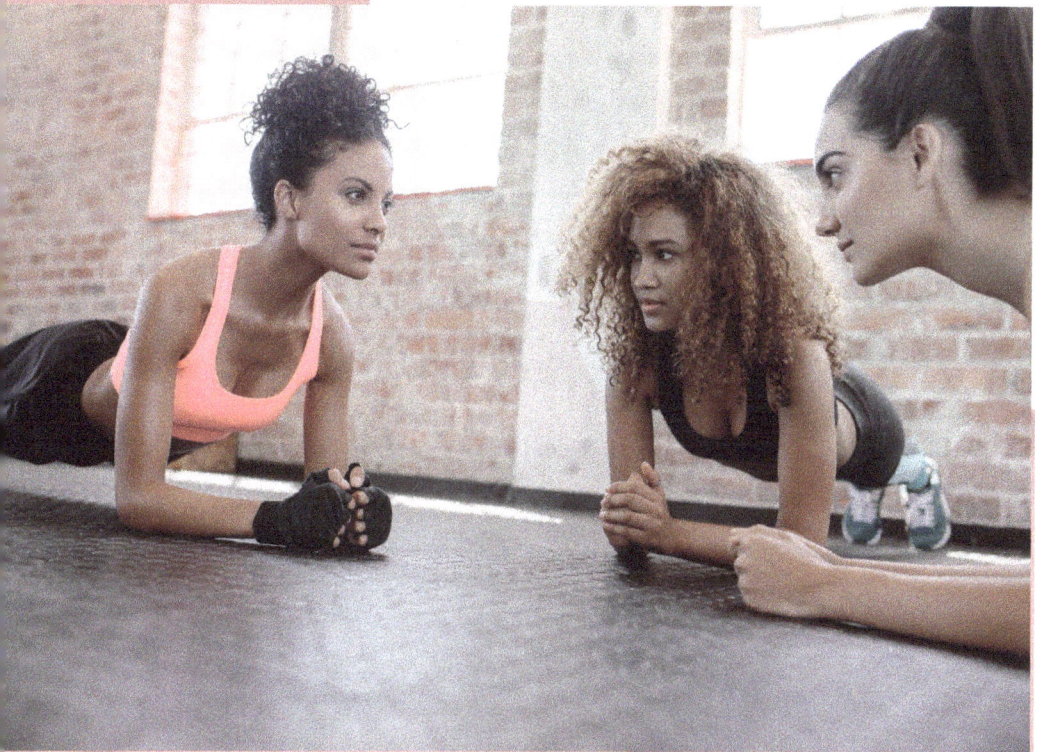

PLANKS:
A great exercise for improving core strength while engaging your whole body. Try starting at 20-30 seconds and then work your way up.

WALL SITS:
These will target your hamstrings, quadriceps, and glutes, start out holding for about 10 seconds.

Isometric Exercises:

SPLIT SQUAT:
Works quads, hams, glutes and lower back.

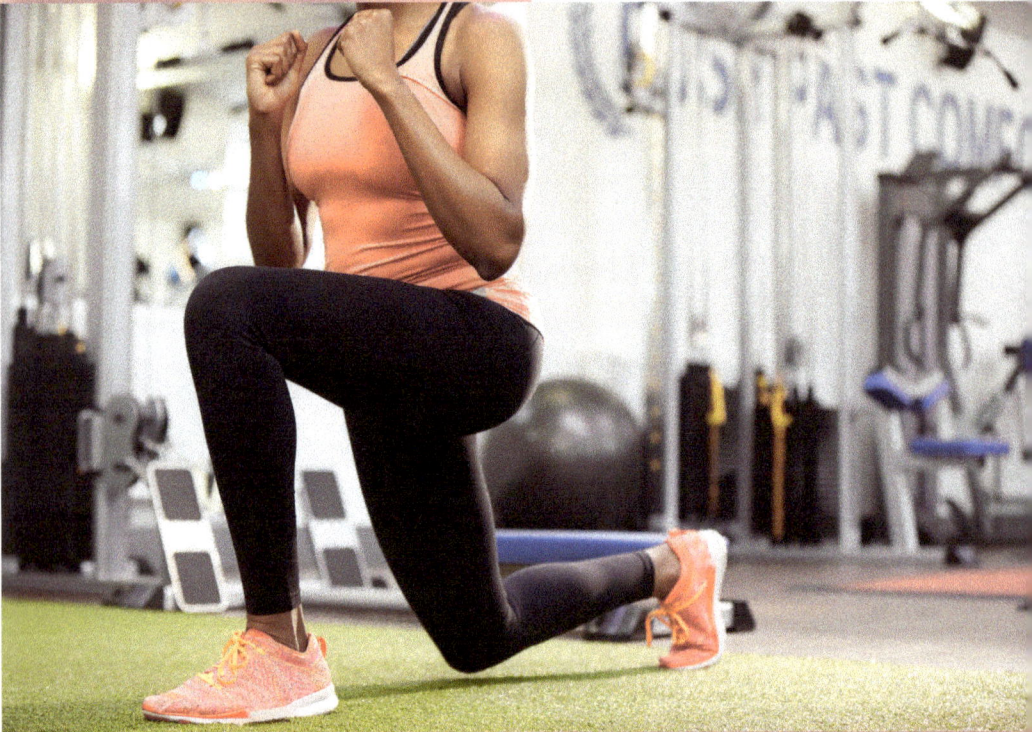

GLUTE BRIDGE:
Works your hamstrings and glutes, start at about 30 seconds.

The Macro Breakdown

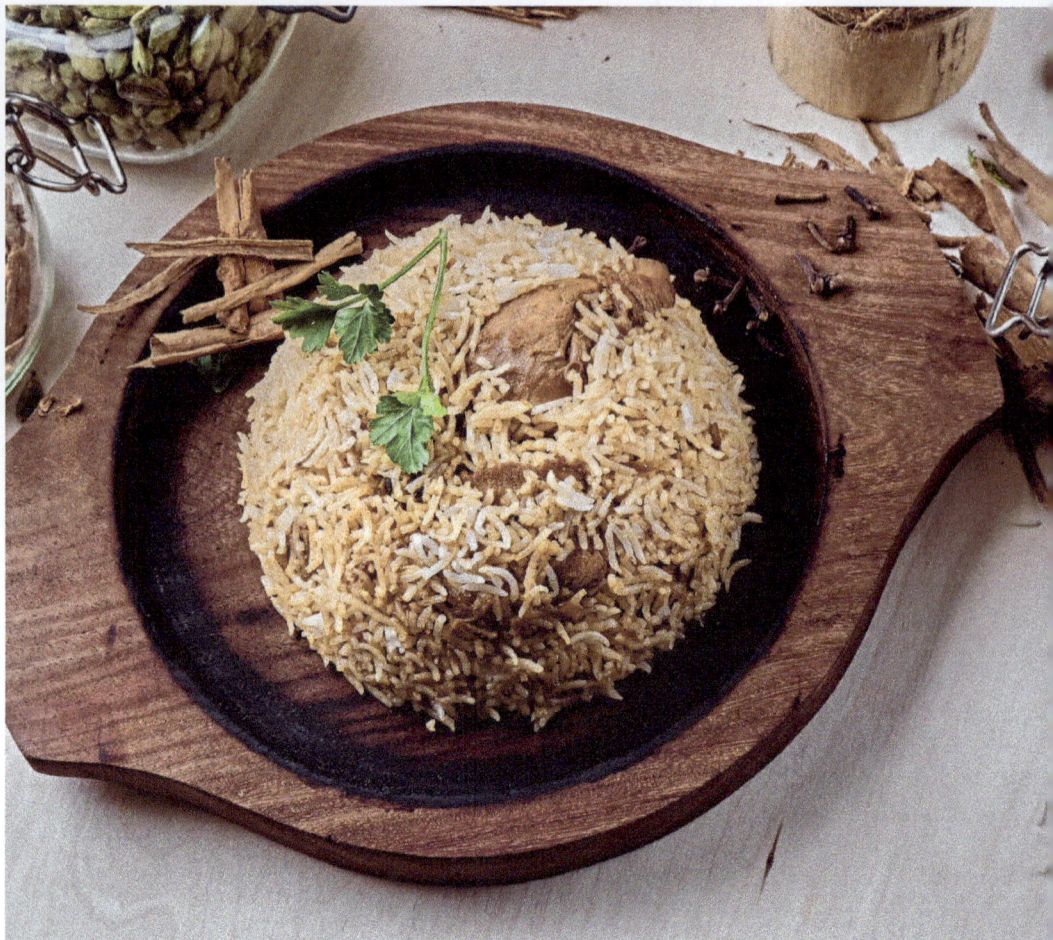

Diet is paramount

So, you are looking to gain size and aren't quite sure how to go about doing that. Most people have the training and lifting down, but you must have a diet that provides the energy you need to lift.

When I started competing, I relied on my personal trainer to tell me what to eat and when to eat it. It was the normal four-week training plan accompanied by the "Bro" diet.

The "Bro" diet excludes processed foods and restricts you to whole grains, green leafy veggies, tuna, tilapia or some other white fish, and a 96-99% lean meat. This diet makes it extremely hard to enjoy life, but some have managed to use it to prep.

Now, on the other hand, you have the If It Fits Your Macros Diet (IIFYM). IIFYM allows you to eat flexibly and manage your diet on your own based off a set number that is calculated from your daily caloric intake.

While each diet has been shown to get you shredded, the "bro" diet is not beneficial for offseason and maybe lack certain vitamins and minerals your body needs. My biggest problem after the show was figuring out what to eat to maintain a good offseason physique. It wasn't until I started IIFYM that I learned how to maintain my desired weight.

What are macros and how do you calculate them? Macronutrients are the main nutrients of your daily diet and are broken down into carbohydrates, proteins, and fats.

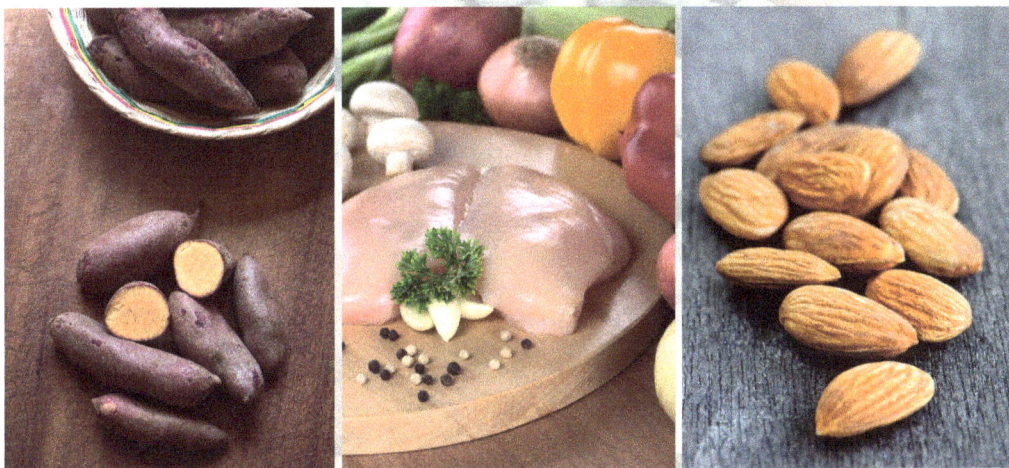

Per Uptodate.com, carbs should be 50% of your daily caloric intake, protein should be 10-35%, and Fats 20-35%. When selecting fats, you want to be careful not to take in too much trans fat at as it contributes to Atherosclerotic Coronary Vascular Disease (ACSVD).

Why is this important? Can I have an example? It's important to understand your macros for weight and health management overall, learning how to control weight gain and loss enables you to take responsibility for your own health and fitness goals. By the way, of course, you can get an example. Let's say that you are on a 1200 daily calorie diet.

Keep in mind that 1 gram of protein and 1 gram of carbohydrates equals 4 calories and 1 gram of fat equals 9 calories. Now you have to break them up into your 1200 calorie diet and calculate the percentage, which we learn how to do in elementary.

Take protein, for example, the recommendation is for you to intake 10-35% a day, so, we will choose 20%. Now you just need to find out how man grams is 20% of 1200 calories.

$$\frac{4 \text{ cal} = 20\%}{1200 \text{ cal} = 100}$$

$$(4\text{cal})(100) = (20\%)(1200 \text{ cal})$$

= 60grams of protein

Setting up your macros can be intimidating the first time you do it, but once you set them up, you can adjust each to see how your body responds and manage weight gain. Now calculate each macro component and increase or decrease according to your goals.

BASED OFF 1200 CAL DIET

Protein: 30g–105g

Carbs: 180g–260g

Fat: 26g–46g

Strong & Weak Supplements

Not all supplements are created equal and it is paramount that you know how much of each you need daily. It is your responsibility to take ownership of your health and check all ingredients thrown your way. I, myself, have broken it down to the very basic ingredients to avoid extra sugars and fillers.

Another great idea is slowly adding a new supplement to your routine so that if you have any negative effects you can identify which change is causing it and make adjustments quickly.

STRONGER SUPPORTING EVIDENCE

Whey/Casein Protein
- Minimum 20g/serving
- Taken as needed to hit daily protein goals (3-6 hours)

Vitamin D3
- 1,000-6,000 IU Daily

Caffeine
- Individual (100-500mg)
- 30-45 min pre-training (avoid close to bedtime)

Creatine Monohydrate
- 5g Daily

Curcumin
- 80-500mg (with piperine)

Melatonin (if needed)
- 0.5-5mg before bed

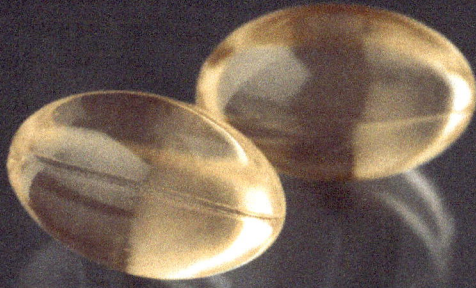

WEAKER SUPPORTING EVIDENCE

Fish OIls

- 1-15g (Or you can eat oily fish 2-3 times per week)

Multivitamin

- Keep low

Beta Alanine

- 2-5g If paraesthesia is a problem divide into smaller doses

HMB

- 1-3g
  - 30-45 minutes pre-workout if using FA form

Magnesium

- 200-400mg

Citrulline

- 6-8g 30-60 minutes pre-workout

LEARNING FROM MISTAKES

We are all on a journey of learning. With that comes pitfalls, wrong choices and at times a crash and burn. But you know what?You can always get back on top again and make a change. Direct your path in life and determine your own destinations. Yes, plural...Where you are now is not meant to be where you remain. Be honest about your past always and don't downplay your own faults. True maturity is in using your mistakes to educate.

-JAMIE JAI

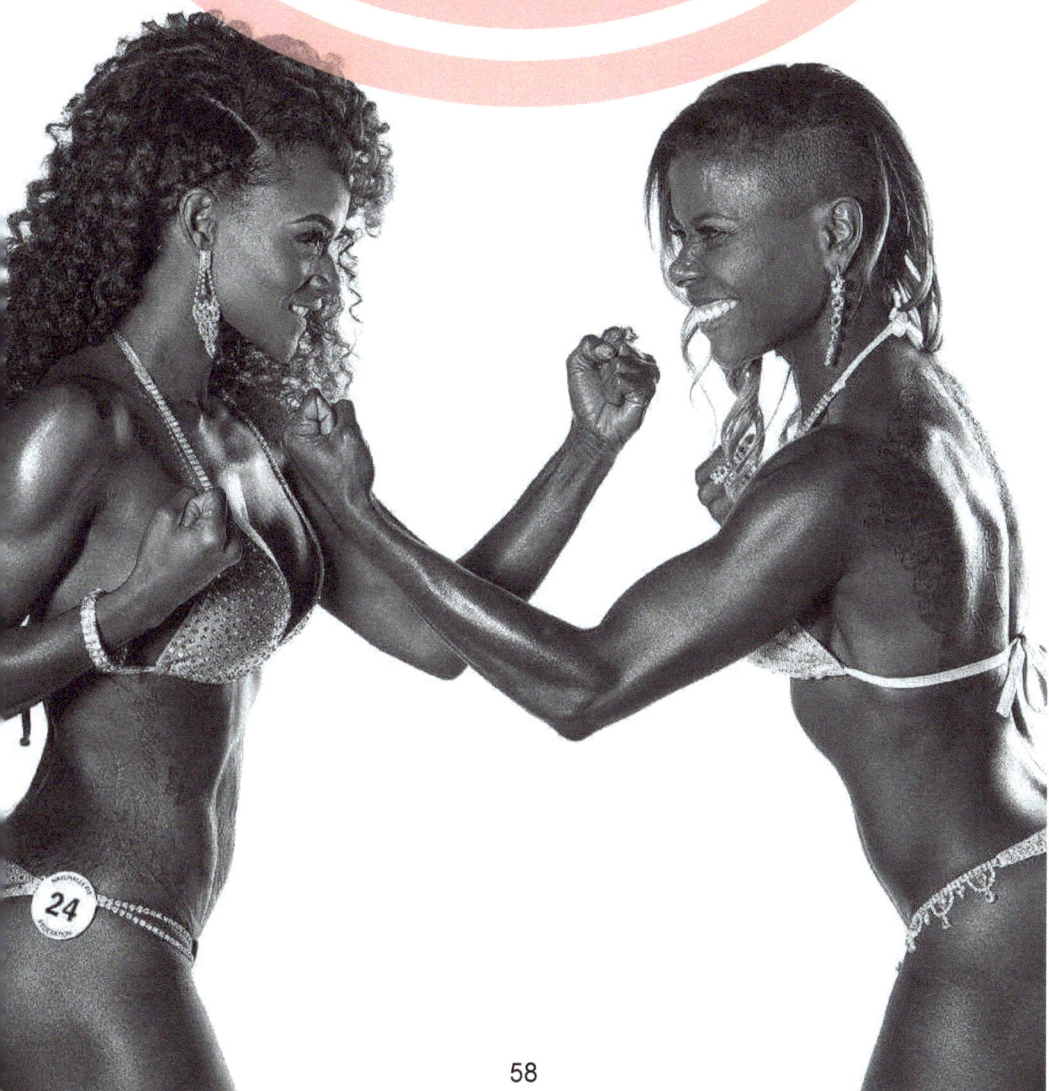

Super Moms

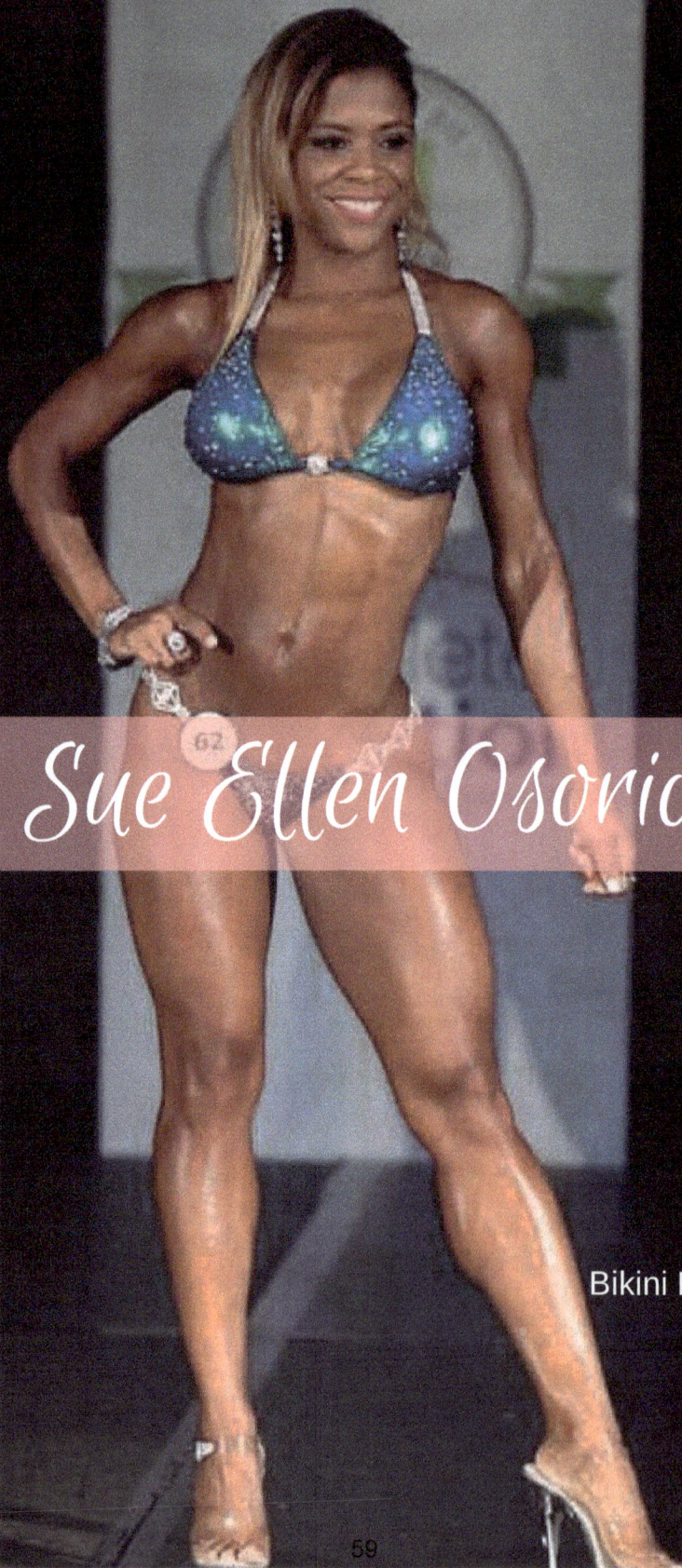

Sue Ellen Osorio

Bikini Pro Athlete

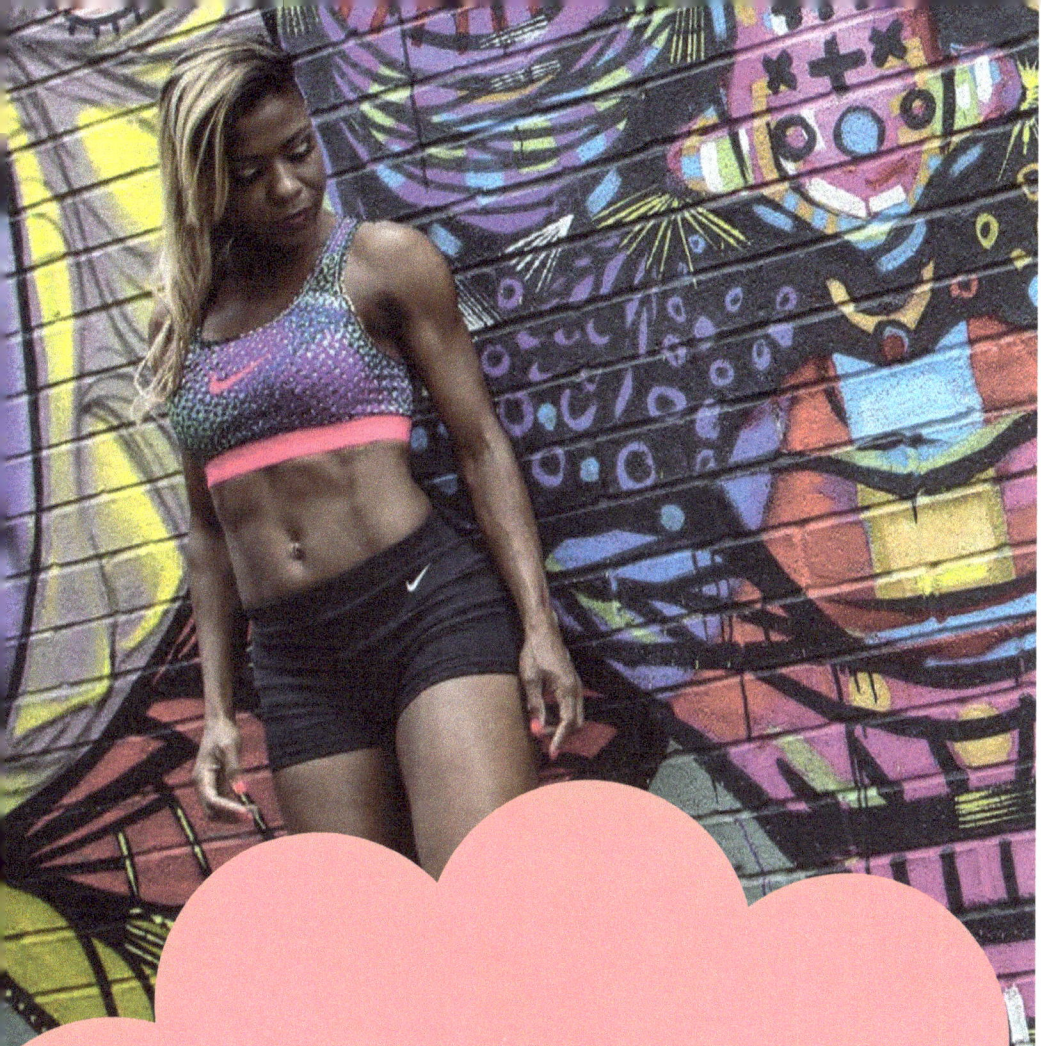

My name Sue Ellen and I am an accountant, a mother of one with one on the way. My fitness journey started in 2015 while looking for something to challenge myself. I have always been active, but bodybuilding was a big change from soccer.

The Lackland Classic was my first show, and afterward, I was hooked. Since then I have competed in four more shows with Naturally Fit Federations Dropzone show being the show that I won my pro card at.

People wonder how I do it. I just tell them I have an amazing group of friends that compete along with me and we inspire each other each step of the way. Also, all my gym work gets done around 4 am so that I can spend the rest of the day working and enjoying my family.

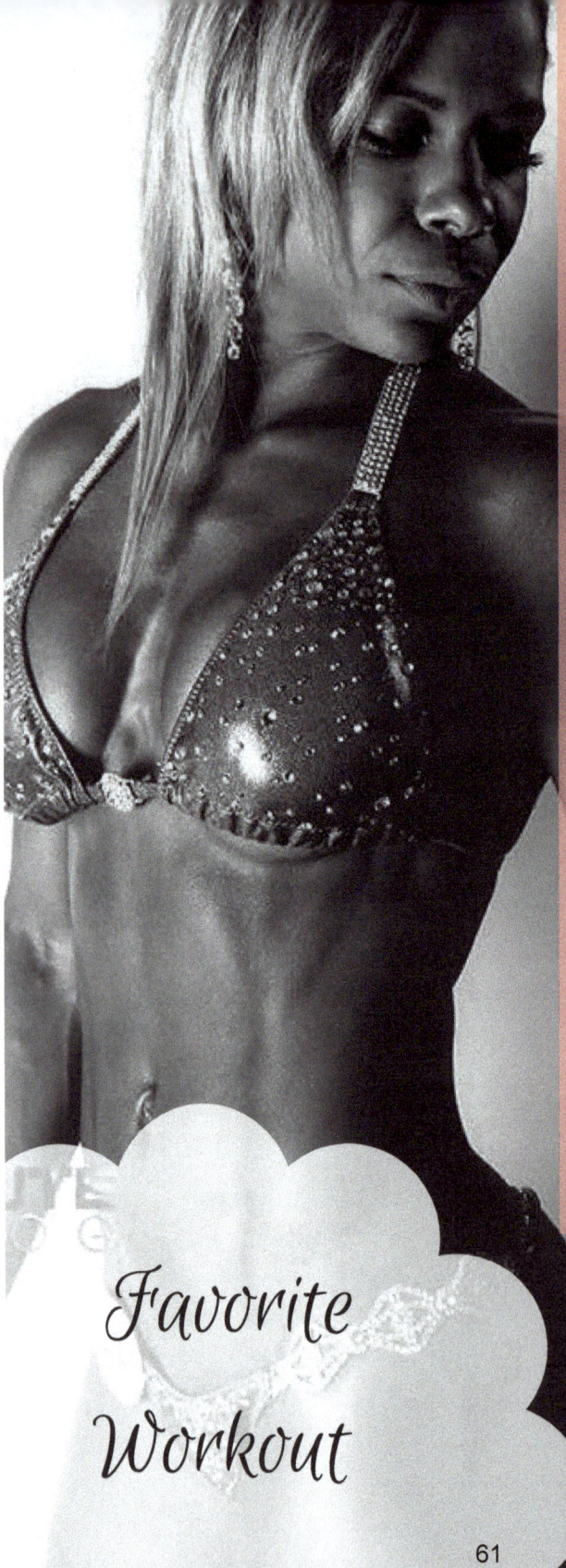

Bulgarian Split squats are my favorite workout. This exercise works your hammies, glutes, and quads. I go for 3 sets at about 10-12 reps.

On the Smith machine, I grab a low bench to keep the opposite foot elevated. While one foot is on the bench, the other one is on the floor planted. Then you would do a simple one-legged squat and rise all the way up. The key is squeezing your glutes while at the top and then come all the way down for a squat.

They seem easy at first, but once you get to 10, you can feel your quad and hammies burning.

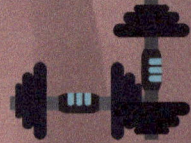

Favorite

Workout

FAVORITE MEAL

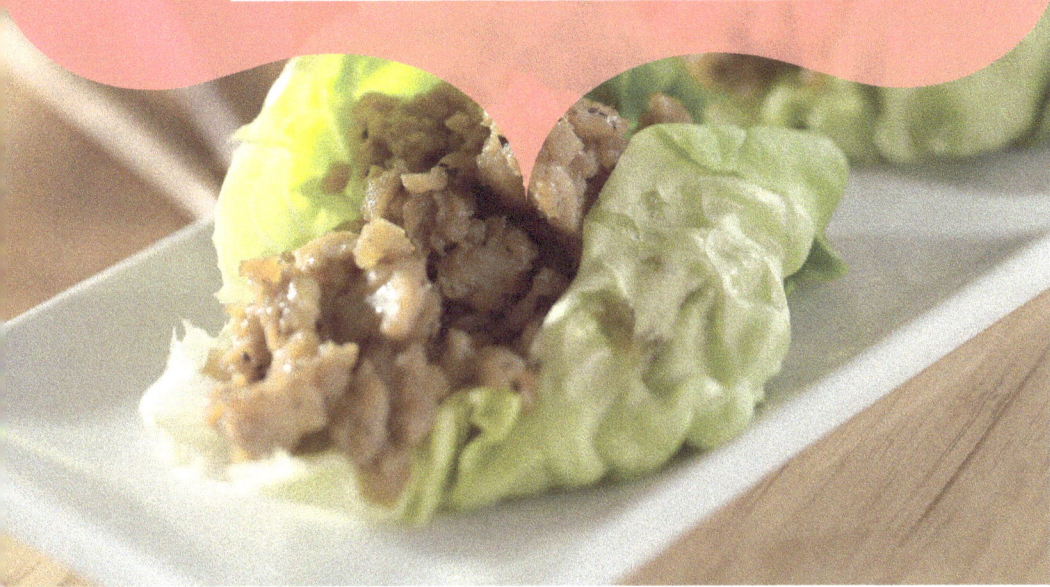

100g of Seitan

2 Lettuce cups

8g Shredded cheese (optional)

50g Tomatoes

Spices of your choice

Protein 33g | Carbs 13.2g| Fats 4.2g

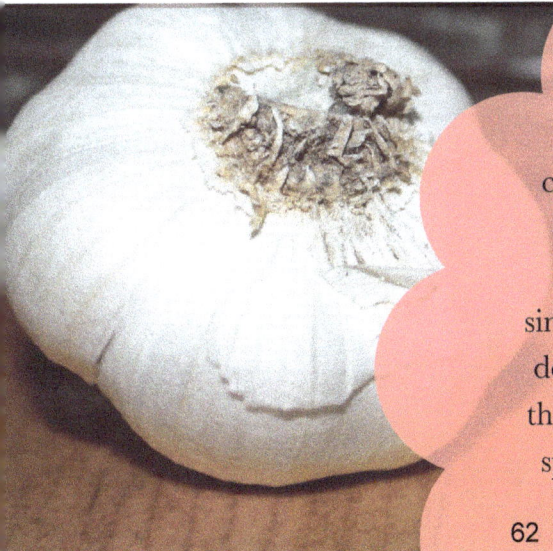

My favorite meal is Seitan lettuce wraps. Cook Seitan in a pan with coconut oil, add garlic, salt, tomatos, and onion (I like to add sliced fresh jalapenos to mine for a nice kick); simmer for about 20 mins. Once that is done cooking all you have to do is put them in the individual lettuce cups and sprinkle some cheese and Viola! You have some amazing Lettuce wraps!

THE MIND BODY CONNECTION

Digging deeply through your energy. Trying to tap into the trinity of YOU. Mind, body, and soul that is, but it's not a trinity. Four factors influence life's code. The body and mind at odds most times, while the soul searches longingly lost. Then an epiphany occurs. Your flesh and heart separate clearing the misunderstanding and confusion the body causes. The most difficult choice we as humans face is choosing between heart and mind. You do have to choose. Learn to align the four, and you learn to take control of your life.

-JAMIE JAI

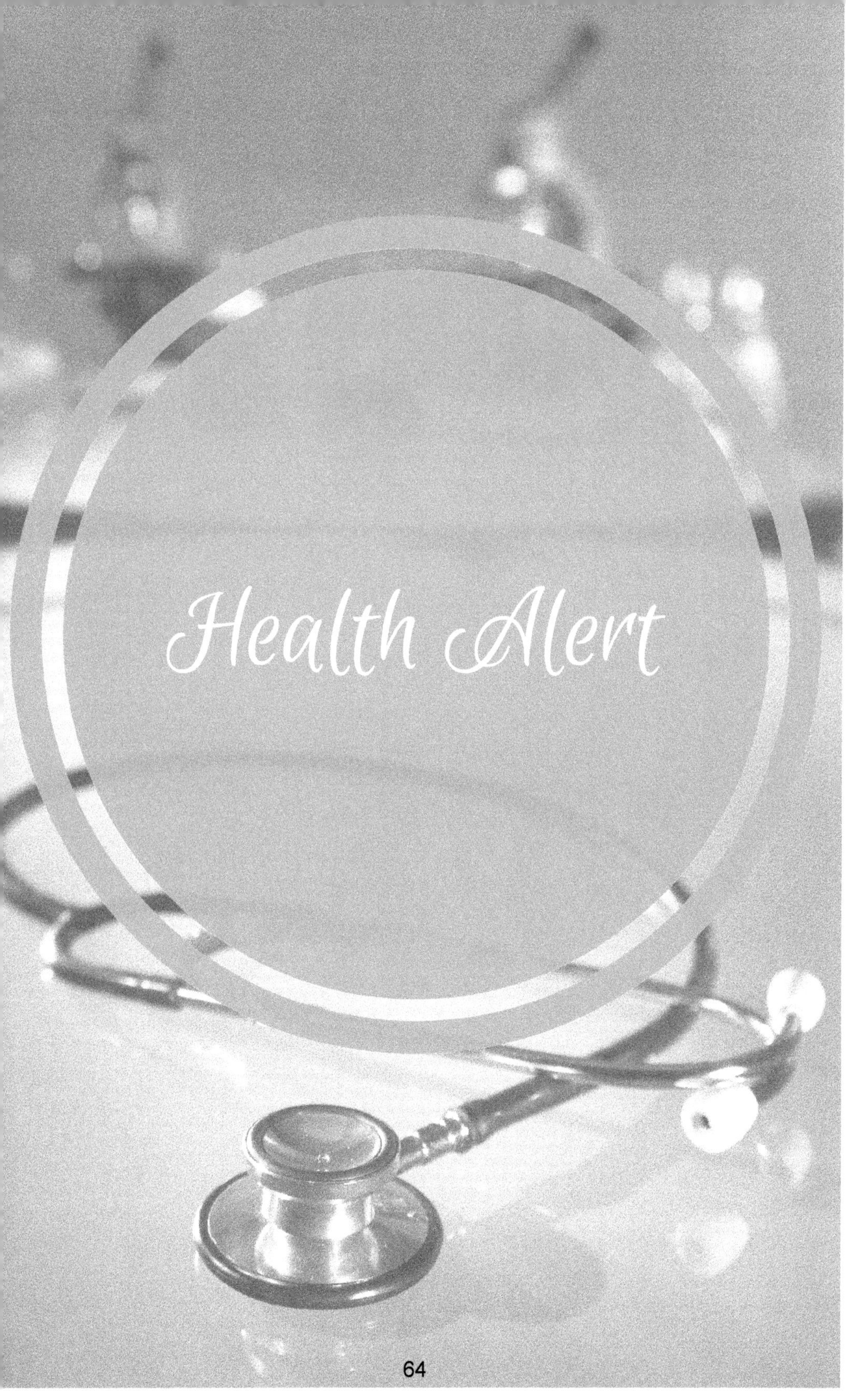

Health Alert

High Cholesterol

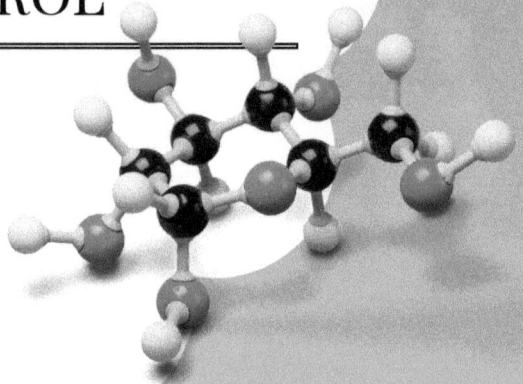

What is High Cholesterol?
High Cholesterol is also know as hyperlipidemia.
Hyperlipidemia is an increase of Lipids, or fats and triglycerides
in the blood. Lipids are broken down into very low-density
lipoprotein (VLDL), low-density lipoprotein (LDL) and
high-density lipoprotein (HDL). LDL is know as the "Bad
cholesterol". Health care providers base treatment off the level of
LDL in the blood as well as your ASCVD score. Significantly
high levels of LDL and triglycerides increase your risk for
cardiovascular disease. HDL is known as the "Good Cholesterol"
and that is due to the fact that it lowers your risk for
cardiovascular disease.

How Do I Manage High Cholesterol?
Foods such as red meat, butter, fried foods, cheese, and other
foods high in saturated fats increase the "bad" cholesterol and
triglyceride levels so avoiding or minimizing these foods is a good
start as well as incorporating lifestyle modifications.

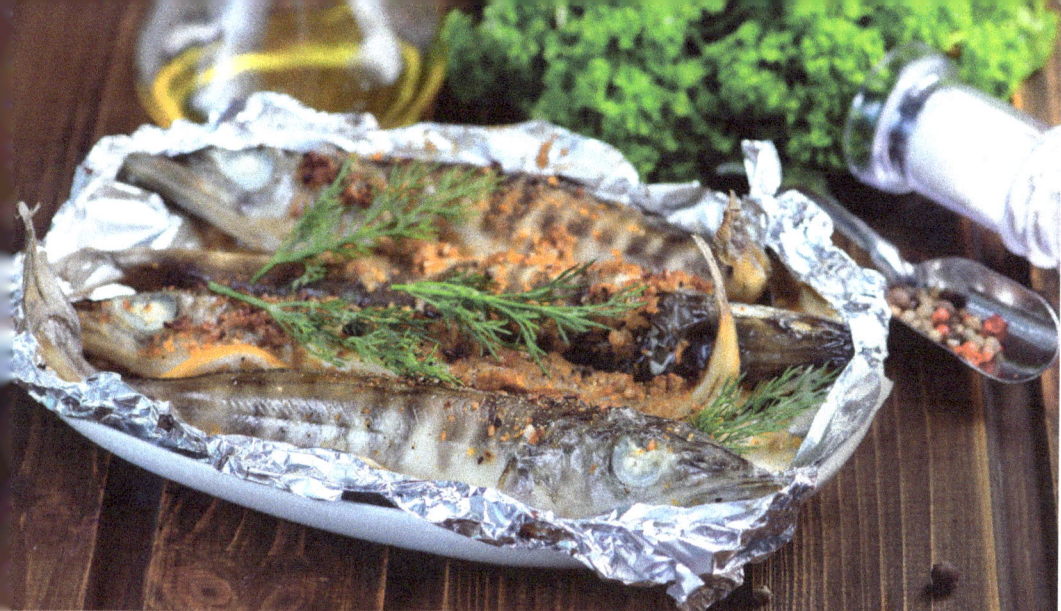

What can I eat to help lower my cholesterol?

fruits, oats, barely, beans and peas are great choices for reducing cholesterol levels.

What foods raise good cholesterol?

Foods high in omega-3 fatty acids such as fish, olive oil and canola oil.

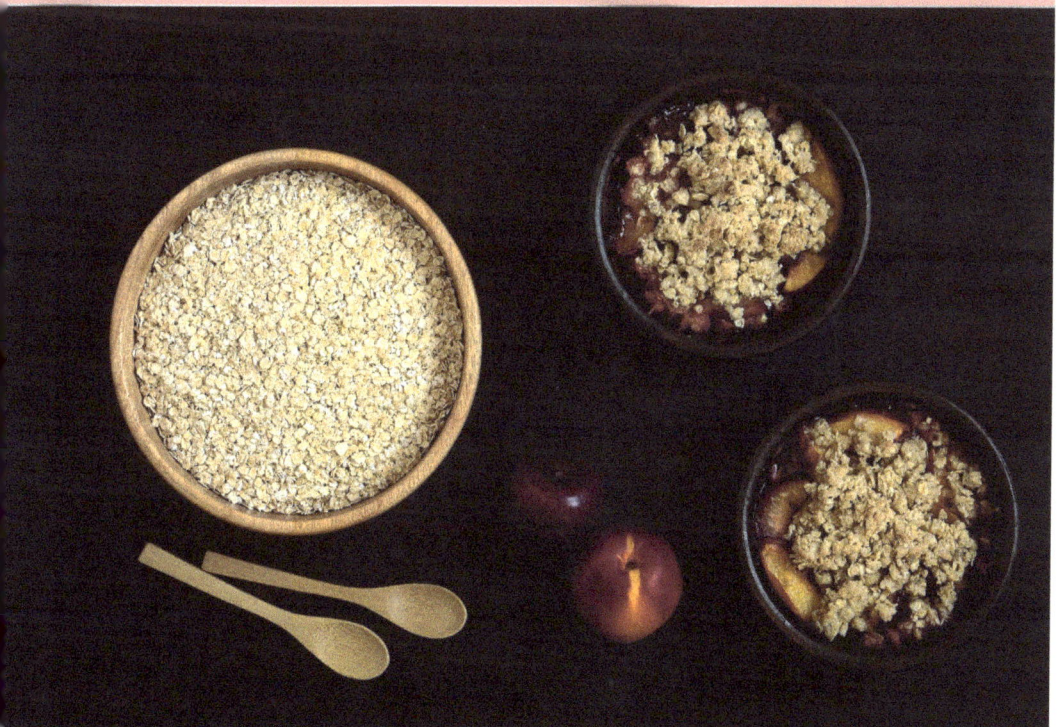

Lifestyle modifications are simply changes in your day-to-day habits. Aside from changing food choices, a regular aerobic exercise such as walking, running and even swimming is known to be successful in helping to lower cholesterol. It normally takes six to twelve months to see the benefits of lifestyle modifications, but if your goal is to reduce your risk of developing high cholesterol or lowering it without medication use then the time is worth it.

Lifestyle Modifications

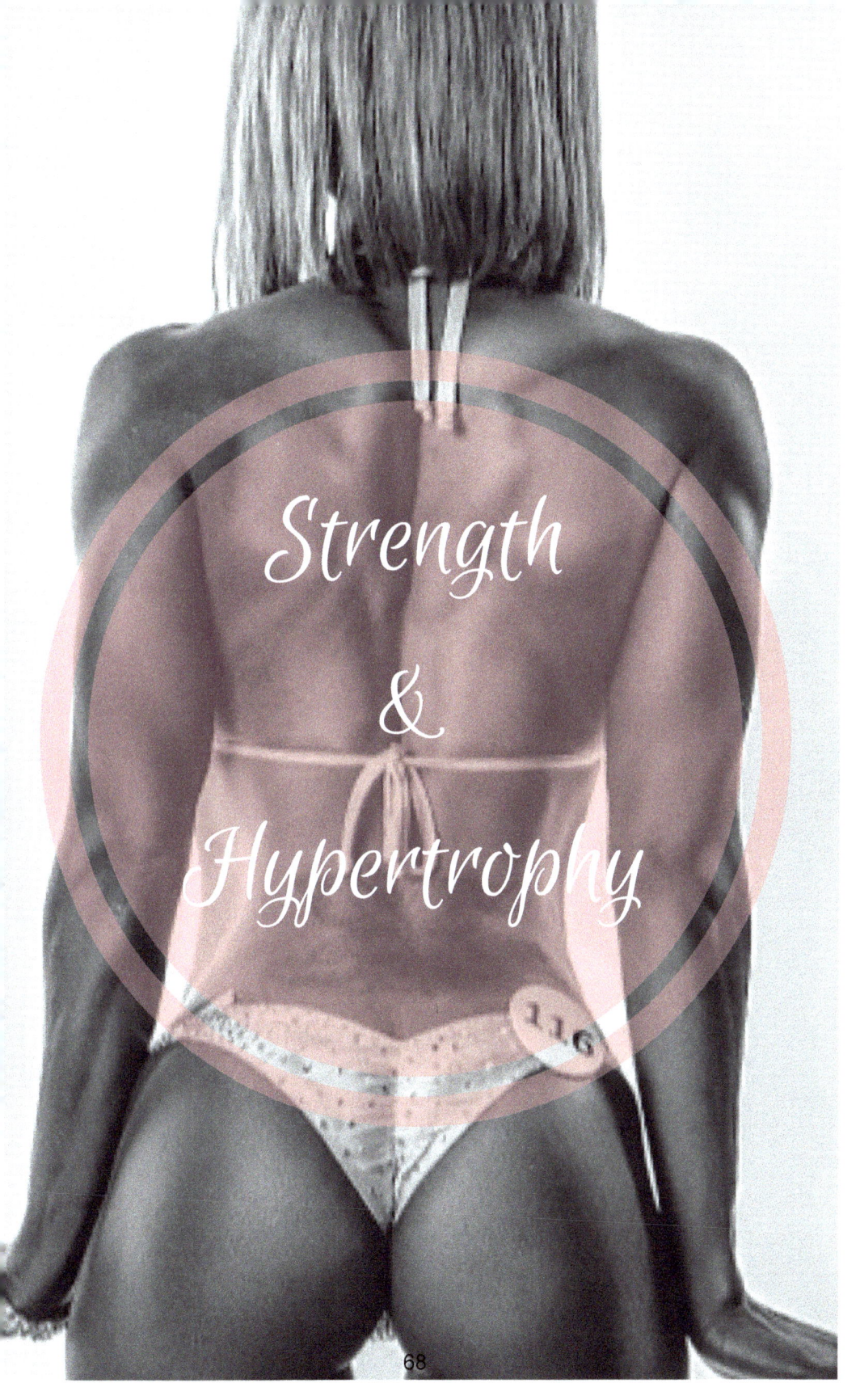

Strength & Hypertrophy

WANNA GET BIG... EAT CARBS!

Many women fear lifting because they don't want to look "manly." Truthfully, lifting weight alone won't make you look manly. What lifting will do is give your body shape.

I can remember walking into the gym looking at the free weights section without a clue as to how to build. I didn't even realize that if I lifted, I could actually get the body I've always wanted.

After years of just using the gym for cardio, I hired my first personal trainer with the goal of getting on stage. At that time I was 40% body fat, and I thought that was great! Not so much health-wise, for my height, that was considered morbidly obese. Yikes right! With determination, I cut fat and then it was time to build.

I've had some diets that depleted me, malnourished me, and ate away my muscle. To do a bodybuilding competition, you need muscles right? Yes, and the hardest thing about it is shredding while preserving those muscles, but offseason is bulking season.
Bulking is time for growth so you need to get in a surplus amount of macros. You need to eat a good amount of carbs and protein, get the right training and make sure you are following a well balanced diet.

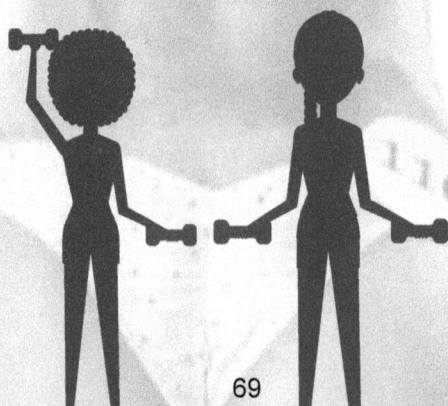

The Breakdown

The Carbs

Carb intake increases insulin levels which lead to fat storage, but that isn't the reason you get "fat." You need to balance your carb intake with energy requirements.

How does it help with hypertrophy?

Well, the increased insulin drives amino acids into the muscle leading to muscle growth through protein synthesis. Carbs are broken down into glucose and glucose is what the body needs for energy. Increase in energy leads to increased physical performance, which equals gains.

Training

There are definitely many ways to train for hypertrophy, but one topic I'll touch on is training to failure.

Training to failure fatigues you right? So, when you think about it doesn't it make sense that if you exhaust yourself before your sets are complete, then your last set will be poorly performed. Poor form doesn't ensure that you are working the target muscle and can lead to injury.

All you are doing is fatiguing yourself, and by doing this, you've made your last few sets ineffective.

For example, if you are going for failure, you do 3 sets and end up with 8, 5, 3 for reps. Your overall total reps are 16 with the last few poorly formed.

Now say you did the less intensive lifting for 3 sets instead and end up 6, 6, 6 as your reps. Overall you did 18 reps with better form. More effective form, more muscle contraction, more hypertrophy.

Bodybuilders love protein for growing muscle, and we know it works, but what is too much? We already know too much protein can cause kidney damage. When we have too much of something we dump it, and the kidneys do most of that dumping. Protein is a large molecule and causes damage as it is being filtered through the kidneys.

Too much protein can also suppress the appetite. Protein is slowly absorbed which means you feel fuller longer. If you feel full, then you arc not going to want to eat the meals that you have scheduled. Most competitors eat 4-6 small meals a day. So it is important to spread your daily protein requirement evenly and ensure you are not intaking too much.

Protein

ONE OF A KIND

Everyone can seek to be anything they want to be, but they can't be you. That's what makes you unique. Take the time to refine and define yourself, because you are one of a kind.

-JAMIE JAI

Recipe

Cauliflower Breakfast Pizza

1 Cali'flour Pizza Crust

4 Egg Whites

15g Turkey Bacon

23g Turkey Sausage

20g of Baby Spinach

15g Syrup

Bake Pizza crust at 375-385 (depending on oven) for 6 minutes then flip crust and cook for another 6 minutes (total cook time 12 minutes). Once crust is baked you will then layer (in this order) spinach, egg whites, turkey sausage, turkey bacon and sprinkle a little cheese on top. Repeat the layer once more and place pizza back in the oven for 2-3 minutes. Drizzle the syrup on top and enjoy . Want less carbs? Remove syrup! To cut the fats just take out the turkey sausage or bacon.

Carbs 20.7g | Protein 39.5g| Fat 17.6g| Cal: 383

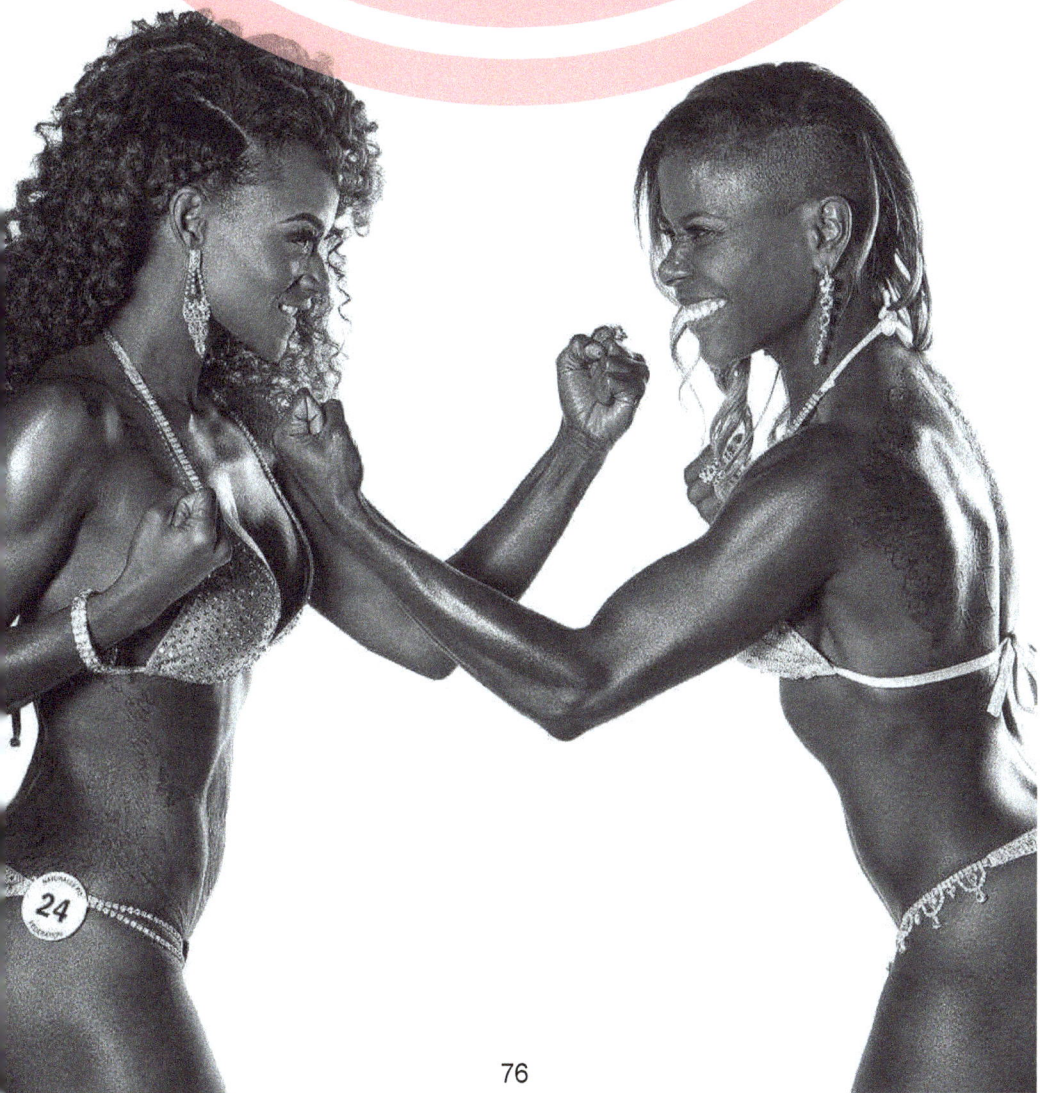

Super Moms

Natasha Thorlaksen

I was born and raised in England. I grew up being very active in all sports, mainly gymnastics and rowing but I participated in all school sporting events. I found staying in shape very easy when I was young. At the age of nineteen I moved to America and started a family. At twenty-seven, after having three children and being diagnosed with hypothyroidism, my body had changed and every time I stepped on the scale my weight was climbing, at an alarming rate. After starting treatment I still felt uncomfortable in my own sk in and sought out a personal trainer. Could I possibly look even better than I did before I started having k ids? It was a lofty goal at the time and mimick ed pushing a boulder up a hill, but I found myself starting to push anyway.

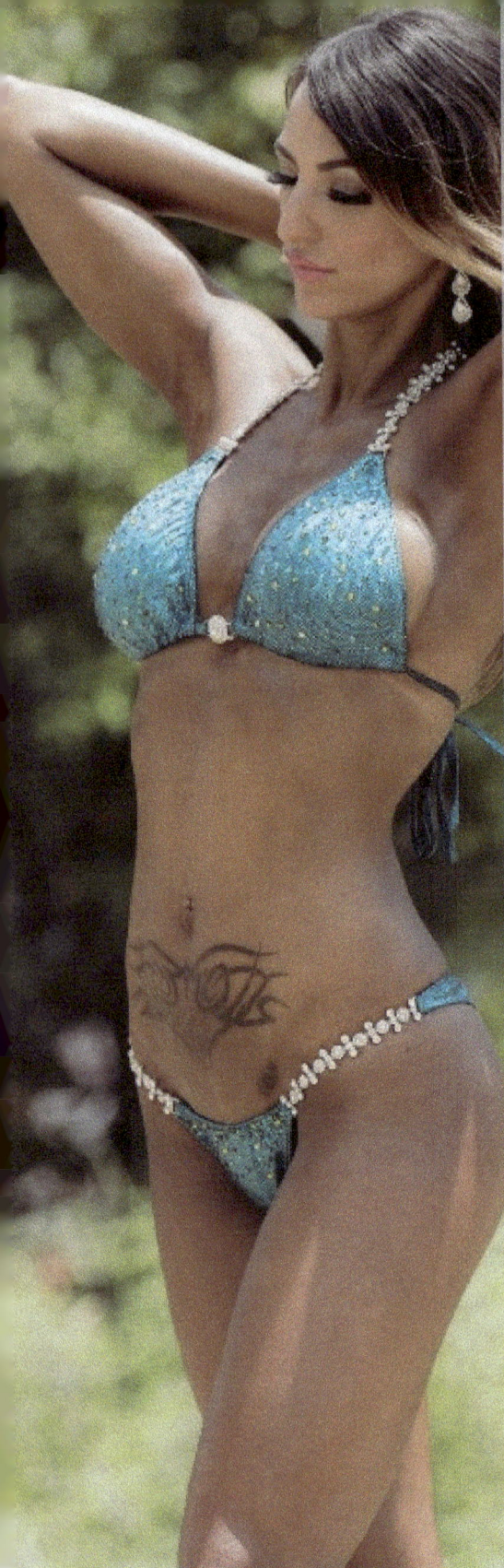

That was two years ago and the group of women and professionals I have met within the fitness world have become my family. Yes we are in competition with each other but we also equally want to see each other succeed. It has changed me from a person who never really finished anything they set out to do, to someone who sets goals and enjoys attaining them. Accomplishment and pride come along with stepping out on stage after all that hard work. Those feelings convey in your everyday life, not just fitness goals and you start to grow as a person. At least I did, that is why I keep competing. Having a job in marketing and real estate, three kids, a husband and a house to run all while competing is not exactly easy. Then there is meal prepping for yourself plus family dinner every night, for the four other people in your house, which can be a little overwhelming at times. After getting up at six in the morning, working, running the kids to their after school activities, making dinner and then going to a marketing event at night, leaves me having to get my gym time at 9pm sometimes. I am tired and don't always feel like going, however, I get my gym clothes on, get in the car and show up. That is half the battle right there. So, juggling isn't just for clowns!! I make time because I have made the commitment to myself not to let anything stop me. Working out for me has become very therapeutic. It seems like the busier my life, the more my feet are held to the fire, the more I want to lift weight.

My favorite workout is the Deadlift. It requires every part of your body. You have to be completely in sync with your muscles, from your head to your heels. To me, there is nothing more gratifying than being able to pick up a really heavy weight with full control. Every time I'm able to add more weight I get excited. Excited to see the growth and progress for me.

Favorite

Workout

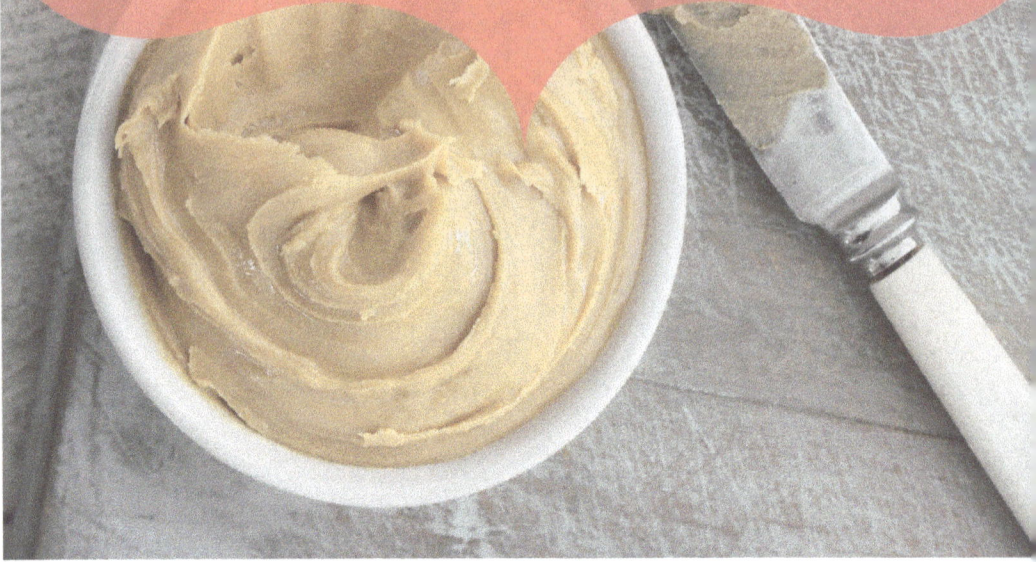

3 Flap Jack Pancakes
1 tblspn Peanut Butter

Protein 27g | Carbs 31g| Fats 11g

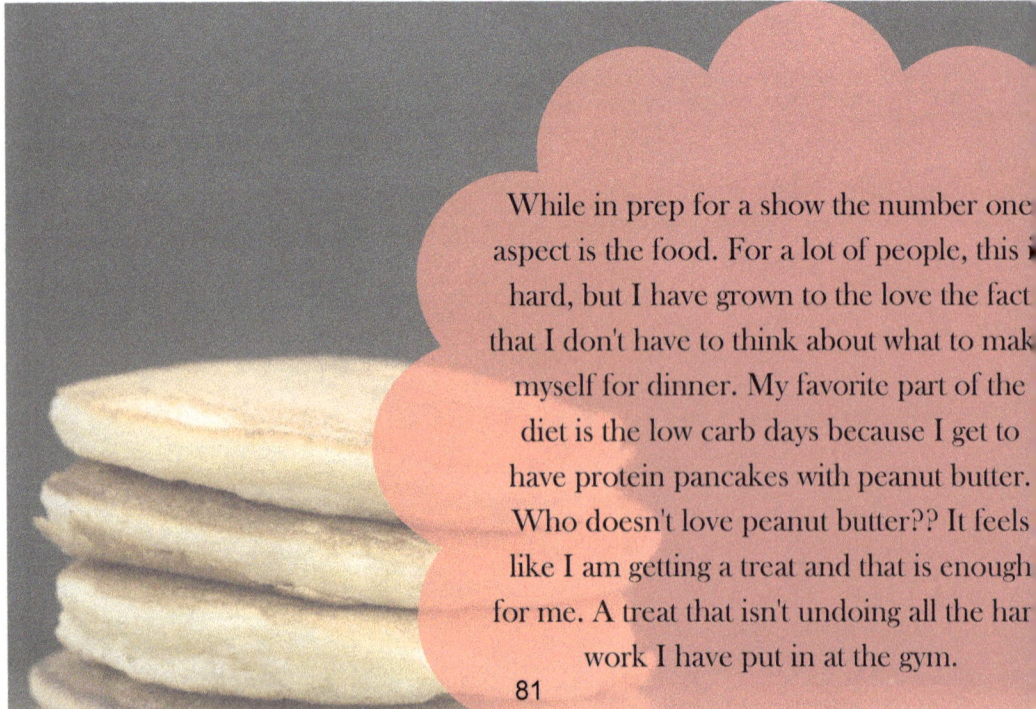

While in prep for a show the number one aspect is the food. For a lot of people, this i hard, but I have grown to the love the fact that I don't have to think about what to mak myself for dinner. My favorite part of the diet is the low carb days because I get to have protein pancakes with peanut butter. Who doesn't love peanut butter?? It feels like I am getting a treat and that is enough for me. A treat that isn't undoing all the har work I have put in at the gym.

ENJOYING THE BEAUTY

It is human nature to always want answers. We pick, probe, take apart and build back up. No inanimate object or life is excluded from this curiosity, yet we still have questions... lack of answer increases frustration making us more anxious for the "why." Puzzled things that seek for what is not yet understood falling deeper in the dark places of the mind. Unacknowledged nor respected beauty all around you, because you fall deeper in love with the "why." You want what doesn't make sense. An undying journey to answers. It is a time and a place for answers, a time and place for the reason why. For now, enjoy the beauty...

-JAMIE JAI

Shoulder Boulders

DELTOIDS

Shoulders can be a stubborn muscle for a woman to grow. I can't tell you how many competitors I hear say their feedback was, "more shoulders". When growing shoulders you have to remember these muscles are broken up into three parts. You have your front, lateral and rear delts. So, when building shoulders, there are certain exercises that focus on each muscle specifically.

Deltoid Muscle
(right shoulder)

Anterior view   Posterior view

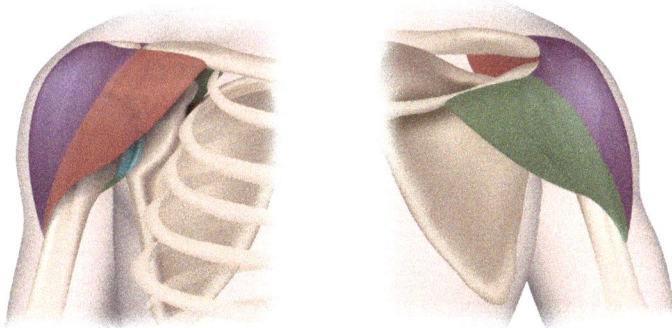

■ Anterior deltoid   ■ Lateral deltoid   ■ Posterior deltoid

Training Them

Dumbell Raises
Push Ups
Cable Raises
Barbell Upright Row
Bent Over Barbell Row
Reverse Fly
Face Pulls
Shoulder Press

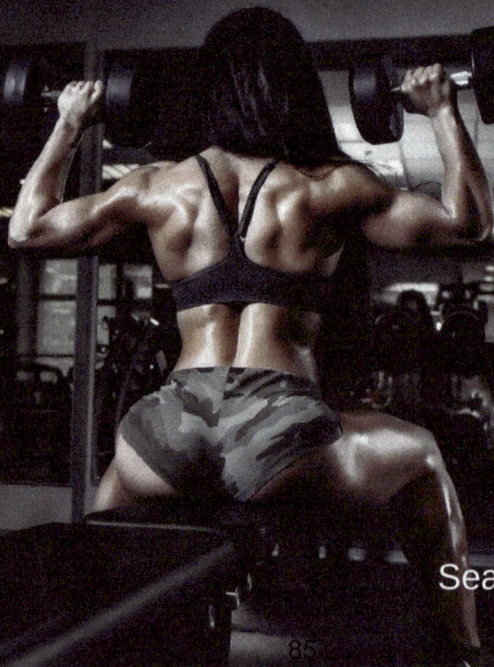

Seated Shoulder Press

Why worry about form? I was once told at the beginning of my fitness journey that lighter weight and good form beats heavy weight and poor form.

Common sense, right? Yea, but there are still trainers and weightlifters out there performing a heavy lift with poor form. When it comes to shoulders lifting with poor form can lead to a variety of injuries. The most common would be rotator cuff tears. Your rotator cuff muscles are responsible for your abduction, extension, flexion and overhead movements.

So, what happens when you tear those muscles? You either partially tear them and have weakened painful motion or a full tear with loss of motion and strength.

For this reason, it is important to lift with proper form. Acromioclavicular joint issues can arise reducing your ability to perform overhead motion as well. If you ever feel a sudden pain, popping, clicking or weakness seek medical advice. Long-standing tears can lead to dislocations and premature joint arthritis.

Focusing On Form

Rotator Cuff Muscles

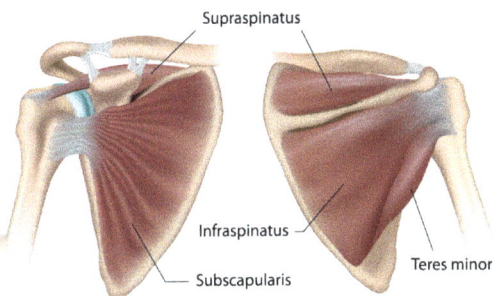

Supraspinatus

Infraspinatus

Subscapularis

Teres minor

Anterior view

Posterior view

Normal

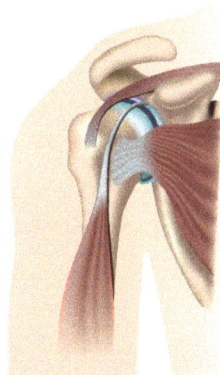

Rotator cuff problems

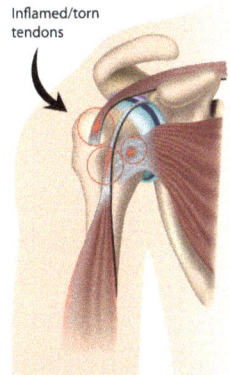

Inflamed/torn tendons

Armageddon

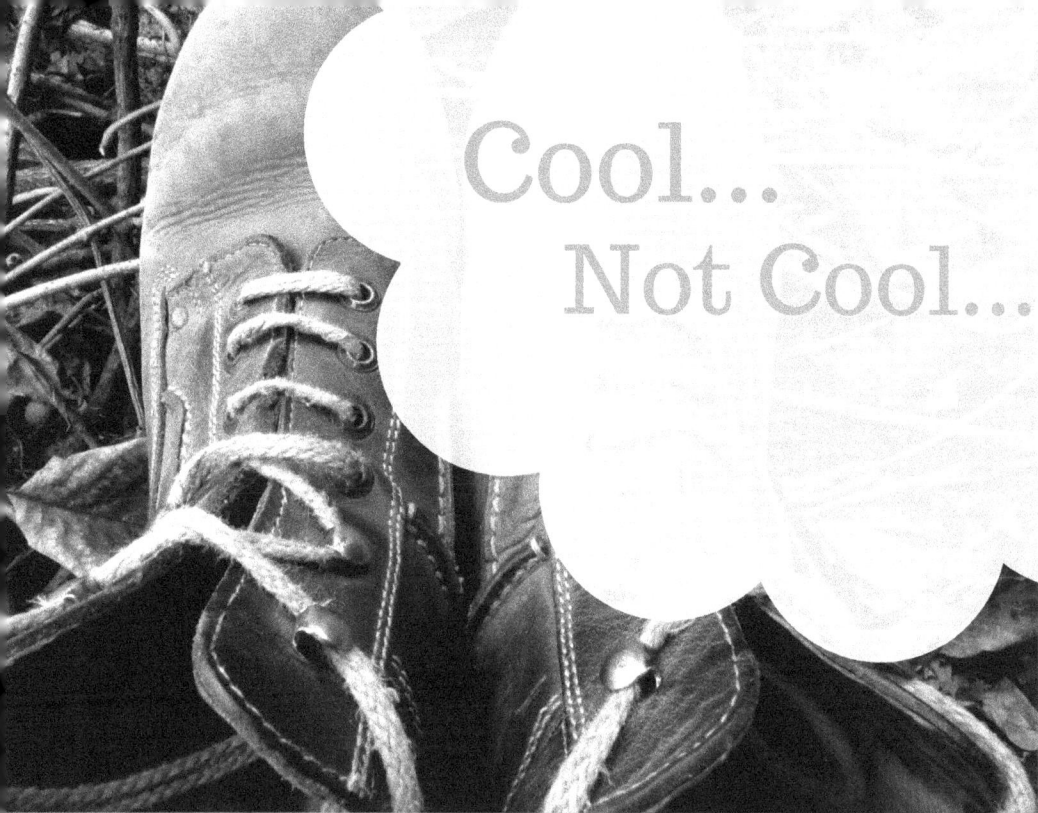

Cool...
Not Cool...

It was 2008, and I was stuck in Iraq. I've always been a feminine woman, but femininity had no place here. The first night I arrived, it was raining and freezing cold. Orders were to report into work as soon as we landed, but there was no way my body could make it out of my trailer. Sitting on a plane the whole flight over was long, and I was exhausted. We stopped several places along the way, but one stop wasn't planned.

I looked out the window thinking that God was working some kind of miracle. It was actually flames from our plane being on fire. We had to emergency land in Canada, and thankfully the Canadians wouldn't allow us to sleep on their airport floors. Their kindness provided a warm place to sleep and three hot meals, and in two days, we were back at it again.

We had a smooth landing that night, meaning we weren't under fire. We got our briefings and were assigned a trailer. The rain fell heavy as the cold tore through my wet boots.

I opened the door of the trailer and was surprised. I shared a trailer with three other women. Now, let me describe this trailer. It was big enough for two bunk beds, four small narrow lockers, and four-night stands.

Some of us worked days and some nights. When you did get sleep, you'd wake up on the floor covered with your flack vest. Thankfully my subconsciousness kicked in during alarm reds, and the robotic me took over. Pretty much there was no such thing as sleep.

The crowded trailer didn't last long though. Women came and went as the months past. All I could think about was getting home, but most importantly all I could think about was doing my best to get those that were injured outside the wire home too. I was twenty-three-years-old at the time and wasn't really prepared for all the lessons I would learn and things I would see. When you're there, you are family.

I didn't even know him, but I felt all his pain and mourning. He came through the emergency room giving his battle buddy CPR. I watched the staff pry him off, so that they could save his life. Two days later we draped his battle buddies casket and saluted as they carried him away. I had never heard the deep, painful wailing of a grown man before. I had to run to the supply room.

I broke down myself. I could visualize the family members pain and all those that knew him. I could see the other caskets and injured that I carried off the Ambus years before during my last deployment. The soldier giving him CPR was the sole survivor. "Why me, I should be with them," he said. A bond that can't be broken is what that was.

Some good memories remain also. I can remember the some of my Iraq patients. Teaching me Arabic and learning about our foods.

The young man, my baby girl, and a crazy but sweet young woman. Most of all This little hard head twelve-year-old boy who had experienced way more in life than most my age back home. He would refuse to go to sleep until he got his bag of Cheetos.

We might not have been able to fully communicate, but kindness was universally understood. All just trying to understand their purpose in life and find love and peace.

My most memorable experience was on my way to the hospital to start my shift. I was walking with a friend when we heard a noise in the distance. We had been there long enough to know that it was a missile. The cement coverings were nowhere in sight, which meant nowhere to take cover. We looked in the sky trying to figure out which way the missile was coming from when the sky suddenly lit up with fire like in the movie Armageddon. Thank God for that counter attack right over my head. "Cool," a Doc said. "Not cool," was my reply.

In those moments you never knew what tomorrow held, but what I learned is that no matter where you are that fact never changes. That year, I saw things few people get to see, things most people don't want to experience and learned to appreciate the little things in life.

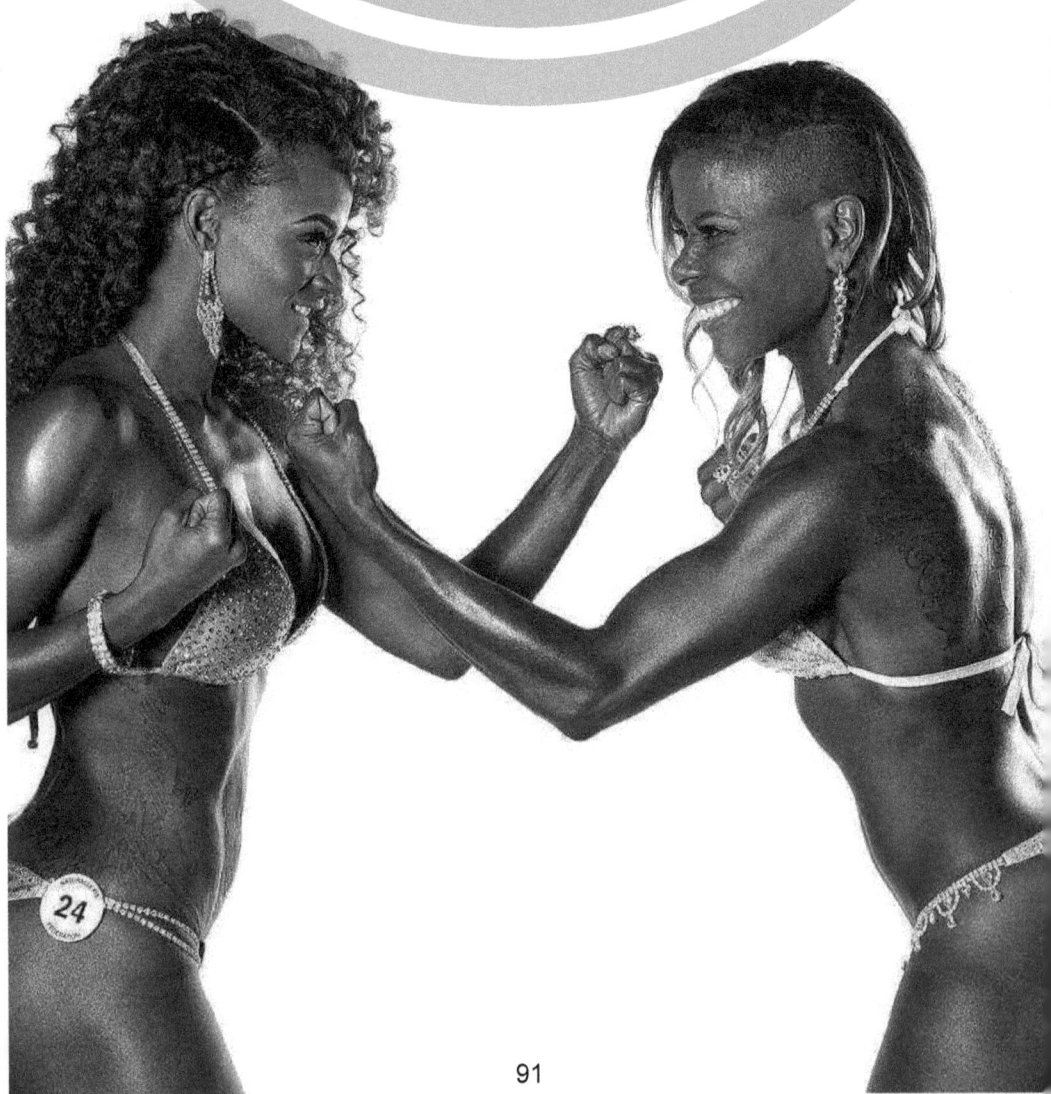

Super Moms

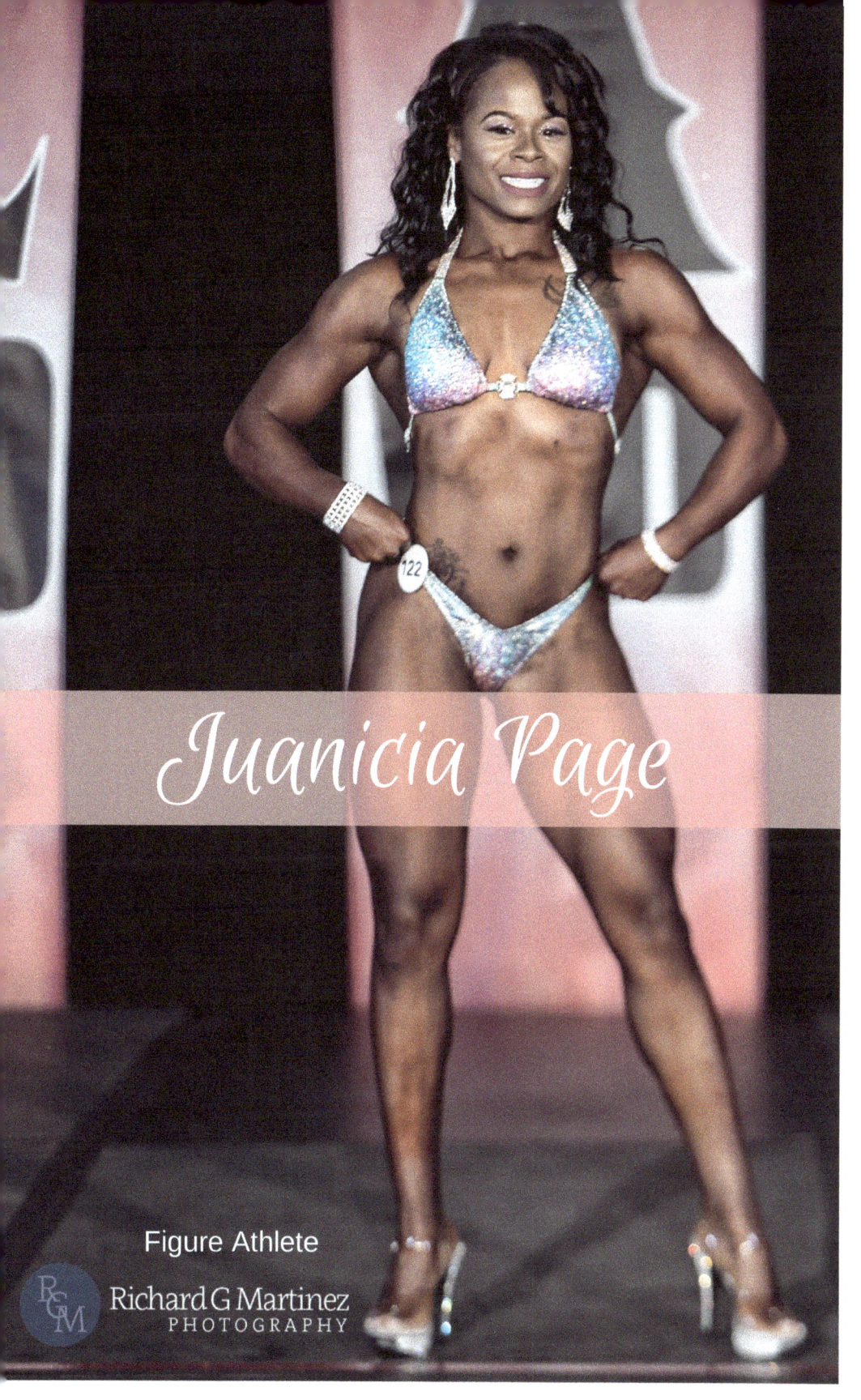

Juanicia Page

Figure Athlete

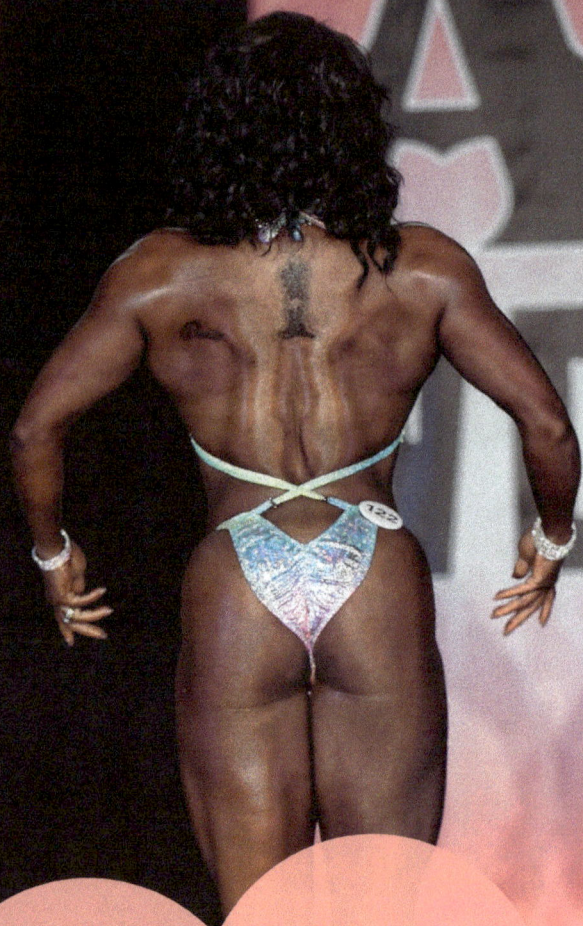

My name is Juanicia Page. I am a thirty-year-old mother to one. I have always been into working out but never knew what exercises to do to build muscle while remaining lean and looking feminine. I never wanted to lift heavy and bulk because I feared looking manly and stocky, especially since I'm only 5'1. Working out began while I was pregnant, but I couldn't be consistent due to my full-time work schedule and pure exhaustion from pregnancy.

Once my baby was five or six months old, I began to seriously work out. I juggled school, a deployed husband, and baby, but still found time to focus on my health. From afar my Husband kept me inspired.

I was drinking protein shakes and eating healthier, but nothing I was doing was really helping me get lean. In 2012 I started to explore the idea of bodybuilding and thought that I would be a great bikini competitor!

Almost every girl wants to start out doing bikini lol but little did I know my body was better for figure.

Fast forward to 2016 when I committed myself to my first show and began working with my trainers!

I was excited to embark on this journey and see how my body would change! I wanted to prove to myself that I could get back down to my pre-baby weight of 125lbs and have that amazing athletic build I'd always wanted. Toned calves, chiseled quads, defined shoulders and a six pack with a juicy booty was my dream body!

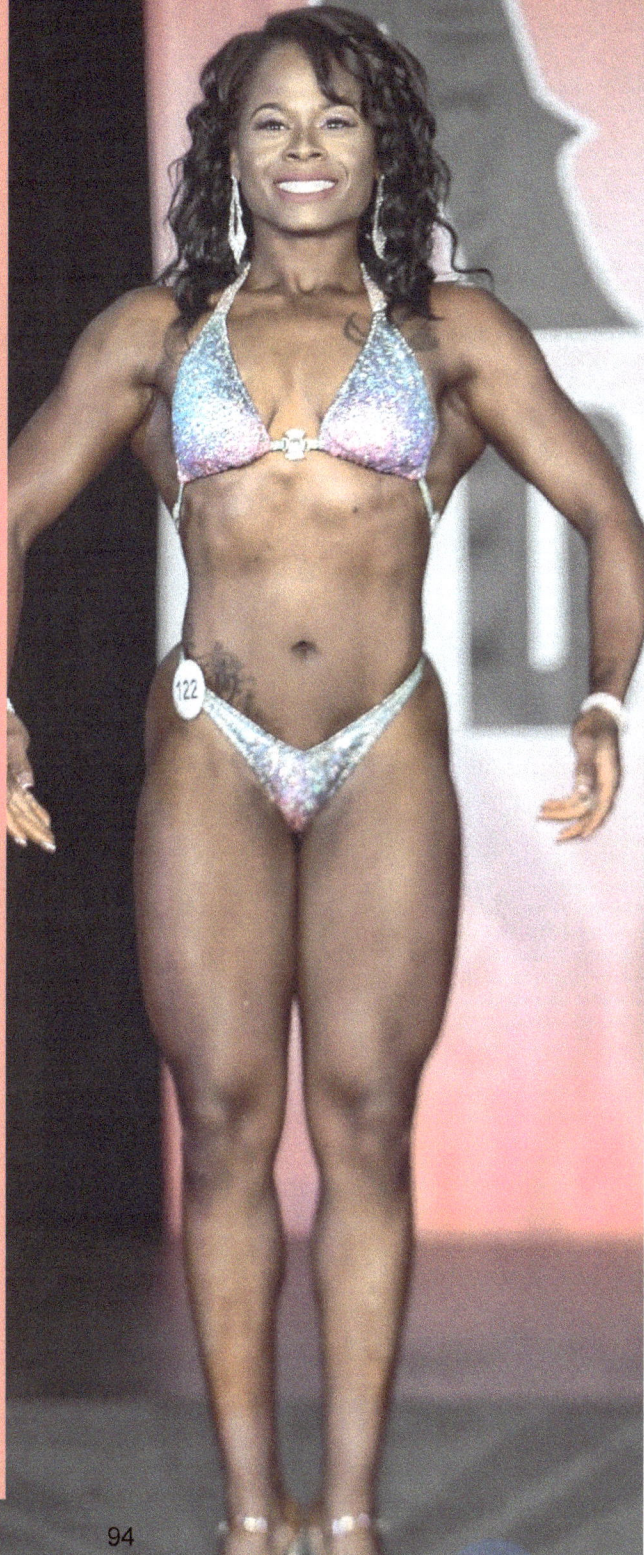

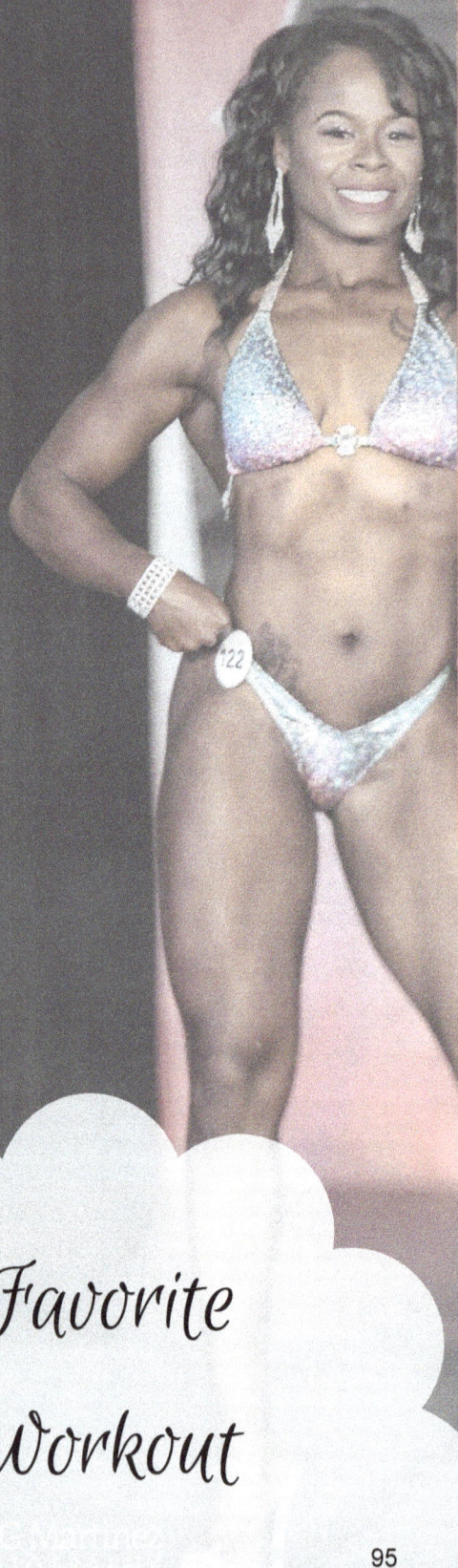

My favorite workout day would have to be legs because like I said I've always wanted a big juicy booty!

I love doing glute workouts like weighted donkey kicks/ kickbacks and glute bridges. A lot of people think you need to do squats to build a butt when in actuality squats build quads. Squats assist in building a butt, but they won't build that but on their own.

I also love to do deadlifts to define the hamstring tie end that accentuates the end of your gluteal muscles.

Favorite

Workout

113g Tilapia
31.3g Cup of Green Beans
3 Oz Sweet Potatoes

Protein 23.4g | Carbs 19.1g| Fats 1.5g

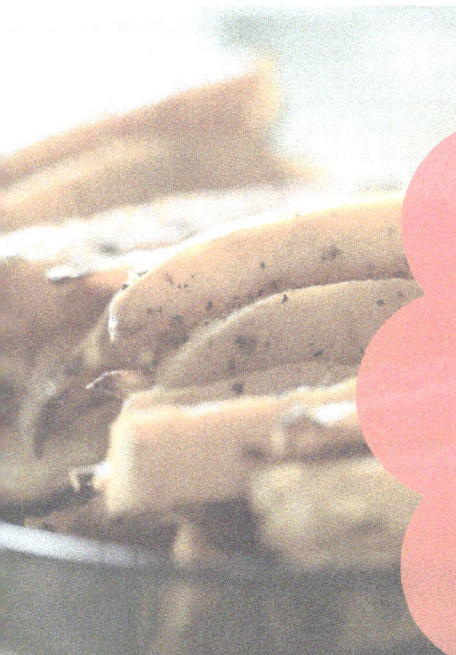

I snacked almost every other day during prep (which is a no-no), and I regretted it! I did have some healthy snacks that I enjoyed while on prep like rice cakes with almond butter and cocoa dusted almonds. My diet food was pretty decent.

I wasn't starving because I had an abundance of food to eat like, baked or sautéed tilapia and green veggies with brown rice or sweet potatoes! That was my favorite meal!

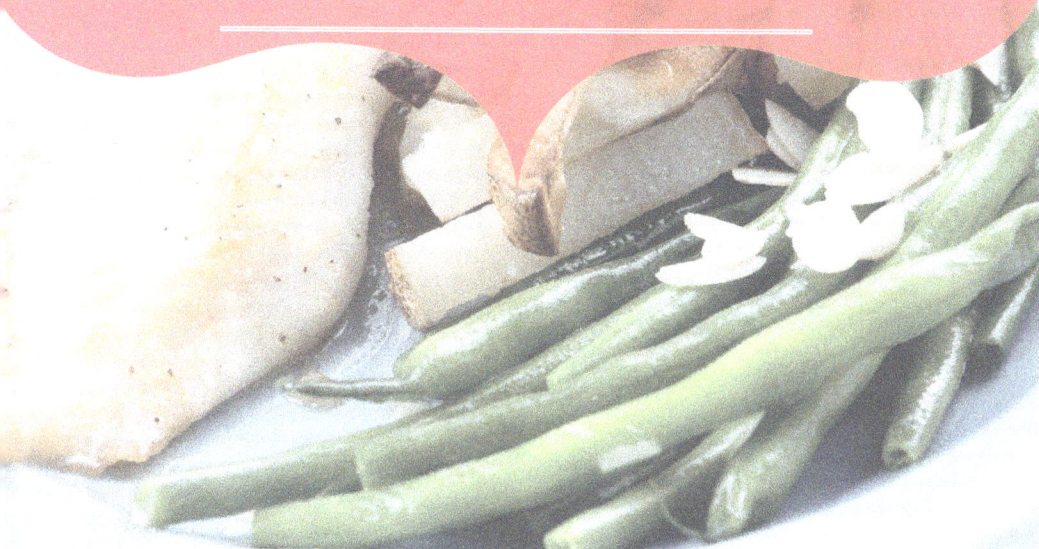

Health Alert

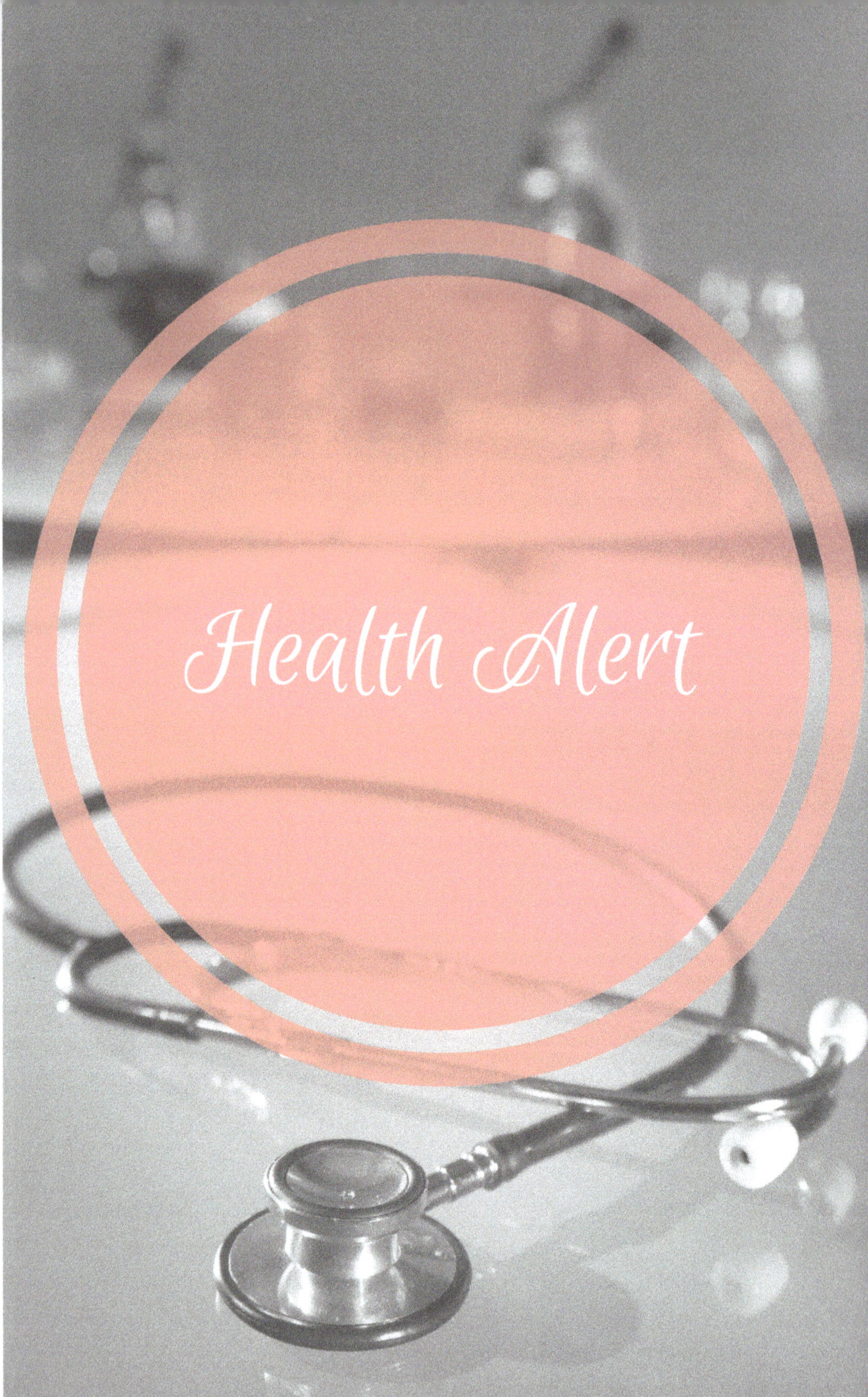

HYPONATREMIA

Hyponatremia is a potentially fatal disease resulting from either excessive water intake or unopposed excretion of the Antidiuretic Hormone (ADH).

In normal healthy individuals, increased water intake leads to a dilutional fall in serum osmolality. This fall signals the brain to suppress the release of ADH leading to increases urine excretion. I have seen so many athletes suffer from hyponatremia due to what we will call self-induced water intoxication.

In the fitness world, water intake is key, and many will say it helps to "Flush your fat cells." Well, it is true that water is very important for hydration, blood pressure, skin and hair, heart rate and temperature regulation.

Your problem starts with lacking the knowledge to understand how much water your body is supposed to intake daily. For a healthy adult, water intake should fall anywhere between 2-2.5 liters per day. Of course, if you are doing an excessive physical activity than you need to replace water loss and will more than likely intake more than the normal daily amount.

Peak week is the point in prep when water intake is the highest. It is very important to make sure that your sodium intake is well balanced to handle the excess load.

For example, Jane is in her peak week and her trainers have her drinking 3 gallons of water Sunday through Wednesday. Thursday until after the show she is to sip minimal water. Not to mention Jane is on a diuretic, fat burner and is told to restrict sodium intake as well.

She does exactly as she is told and after her show, she downs water due to dehydration thirst and has her first cheat meal. Jane drinks and enjoys the rest of the night with her friends and wakes up Sunday with a little extra subcutaneous jiggle which she pays no mind. She then returns to her pre-prep diet and notices that she gains 20 pounds in a week.

What Jane doesn't realize is the extra jiggle is extracellular water due to water retention. She then notices her skin is tight and she feels like she is full of water. Jane also notices she isn't using the restroom as much as she used to and is more forgetful and is having increased frequency with headaches.

After three months of failing to lose the excess pounds with her trainer, Jane seeks medical attention. Jane's doctor tells her that her liver function is low and her kidneys are showing signs of failure. Jane's condition is a result of self-induced water intoxication. She was a young healthy adult, and this was her first fitness competition. The most important thing to take from Jane's story is understanding how important water and electrolyte balance is for your body and the fatal complications that can result from hyponatremia.

Signs & Symptoms

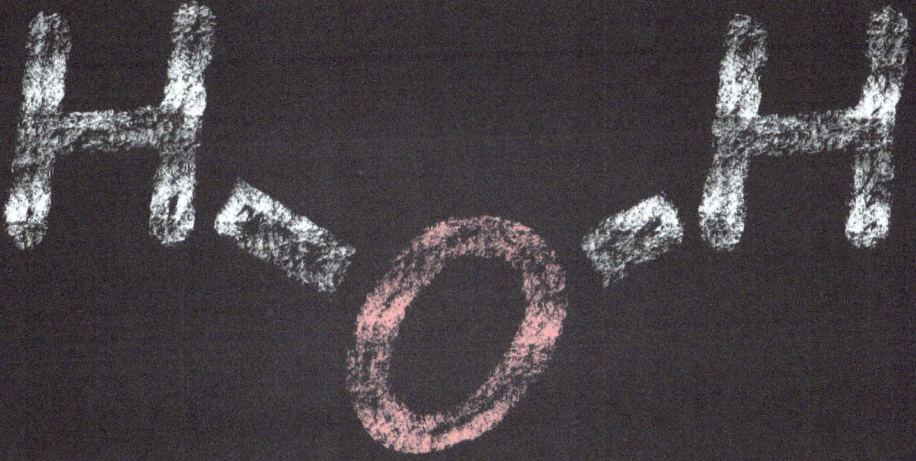

H-O-H

Water Retention

Respiratory Distress

Fatal Cerebral Edema

Seizures

Nausea & Vomiting

Headache

Eating Mentally

Being pleasing to the eye can be a lot of pressure. Every individual has their own body goals, but things get complicated when you start to turn to unhealthy habits to meet your desired body image. Plastic surgery is a whole other discussion in its self.

One of the most common complications among individuals with extreme body idealism due to modeling or bodybuilding is eating disorders. Yes, I said it; I spilled the beans.

Now, craving things can also be a sign of your body lacking certain nutrients and vitamins as well. My best advice would be to always consult a nutritionist or a personal trainer with a certification in nutrition to ensure you are getting a balanced diet.

The key is to being aware of your habits and if you find yourself drifting off into unhealthy eating habits seek help.

Healthy Mental Eating

Anorexia Nervosa

With this eating disorder your tend to restrict caloric intake far below healthy requirements.

Two Types

1. Restrictive
2. Binge eating or Purging type

The Most Common Types

BULIMIA NERVOSA

Eating, in a discrete period of time a larger than normal amount of food followed by self-induced vomiting, misuse of laxatives, diuretics, or other medications, fasting or excessive exercise

PICA

PICA is a commonly ignored eating disorder characterized by eating paper, soap, cloth, hair, string, wool, soil, chalk, talcum powder, paint, gum, metal, pebbles, charcoal or coal, ash, clay, starch, or even ice.

Eating items like these can be your bodies way of letting you know that something isn't right and you might be deficient in some major nutrients.

At the end of the day, you have to understand that none of the eating disorders above are going to help you build or maintain muscle. Your body will turn on its self and use your muscles for nutrients instead.

If you find yourself-deviating from your diet or macros its ok. Tomorrow is a new day, and there are ways to adjust to get back on track without resorting to unhealthy measures.

BMI & BODY FAT PERCENTAGE

<18.5	◆Below Normal Weight
18.5-25	◆Normal Weight
25-30	◆Over Weight
30-35	◆Class I Obesity
35-40	◆Class II Obesity
40+	◆Class III Obesity

BMI stands for Body Mass Index. BMI is used to check your weight in kilogram per square meter, so you are looking at the amount of mass you have for your height. This can be used to calculate whether or not you are carrying the right amount of weight for your frame. BMI alone will not tell you body fat. This means that you can be over or underweight even if you are solid muscle.

Weight just doesn't pertain to fat. You can be majority muscle and have a high BMI leading to additional strain on your joints as well as strain on your heart. Your heart has to work harder to get blood to these areas, and your joints are only made to withstand so much weight before wear and tear occur. All possibly leading to premature heart failure and osteoarthritis.

FEMALE BODY FAT % COMPARISONS

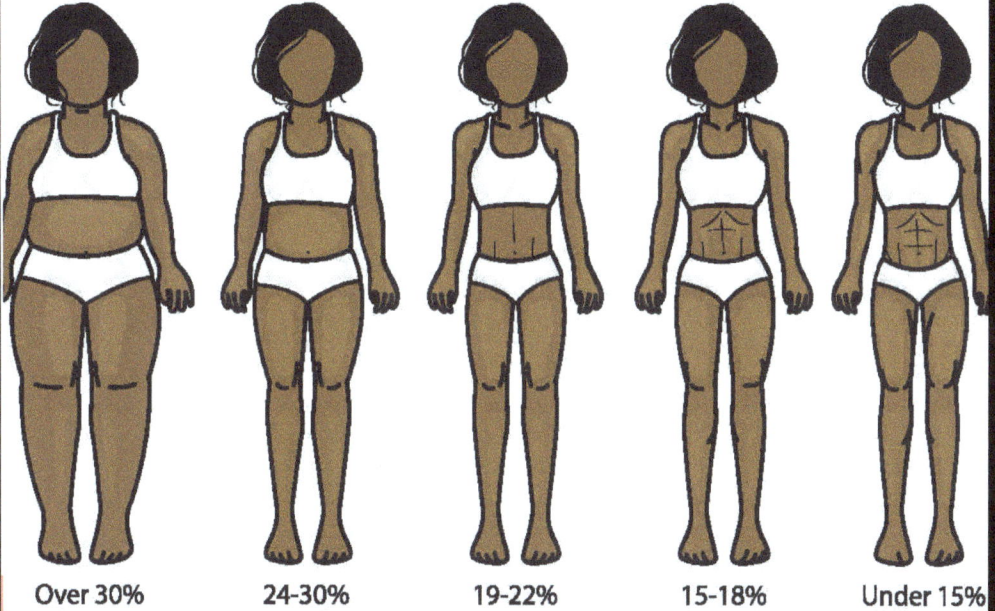

| Over 30% | 24-30% | 19-22% | 15-18% | Under 15% |

Lower Body Fat % = Majority of scale weight is lean tone and low in fat
Higher Body Fat % = Majority of scale weight is fat less lean tone

Body Fat percentage is obtained from a set of measurements such as those from your arms, bust, bra line, navel, hip, glutes, and thighs. There are several different calculators you can look up online or apps you can download that will help you get a good idea of your fat percentage and BMI. With these two measurements together you can monitor weight and fat percent.

Healthy for you and your body doesn't mean you have to sacrifice good foods or competition goals. Notice in the picture that abs appear around 15-18% body fat. On a macro diet, you can manage that.

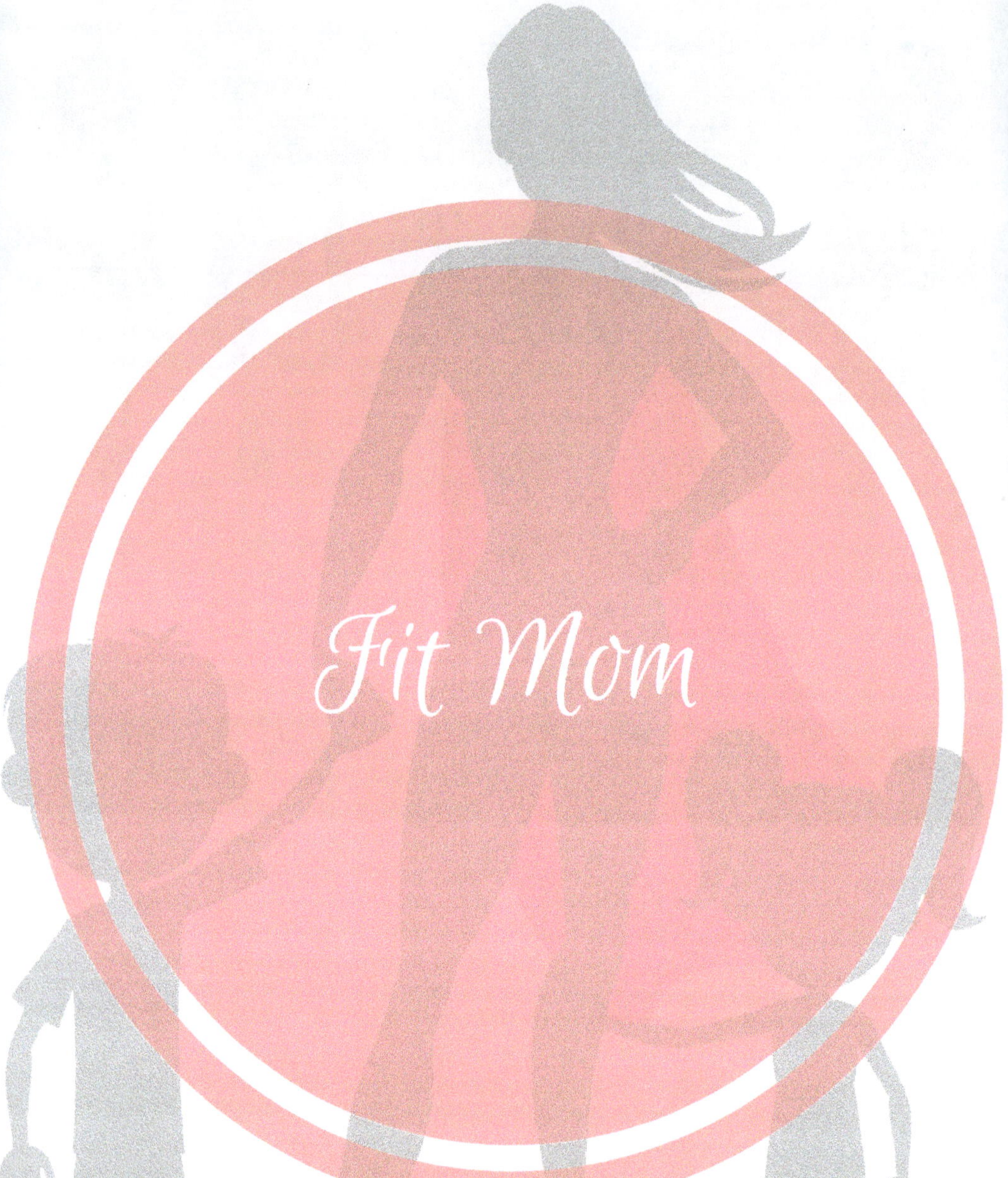

Fit Mom

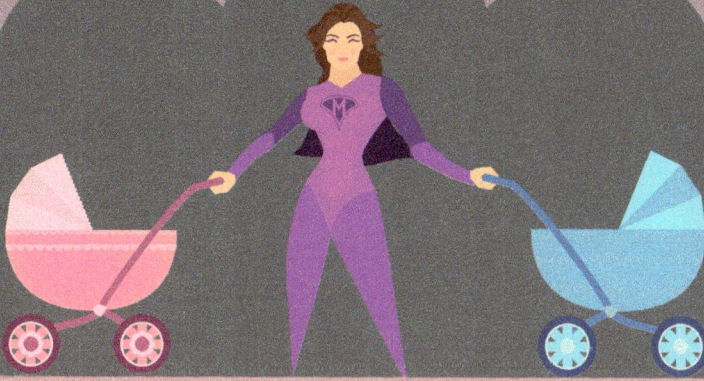

In a time where juggling work and kids can leave a mom feeling overworked, spread thin, and lacking time to nurture herself we must remember it is ok to have moments of selfishness. You must take time out for your own mental, emotional, and the most neglected, physical health.

Your children are looking up to you and learning from you how to balance all areas of life. So, teach them well. Show them how to navigate under pressure. Make no excuses and remember they are always watching.

NO EXCUSES!!!

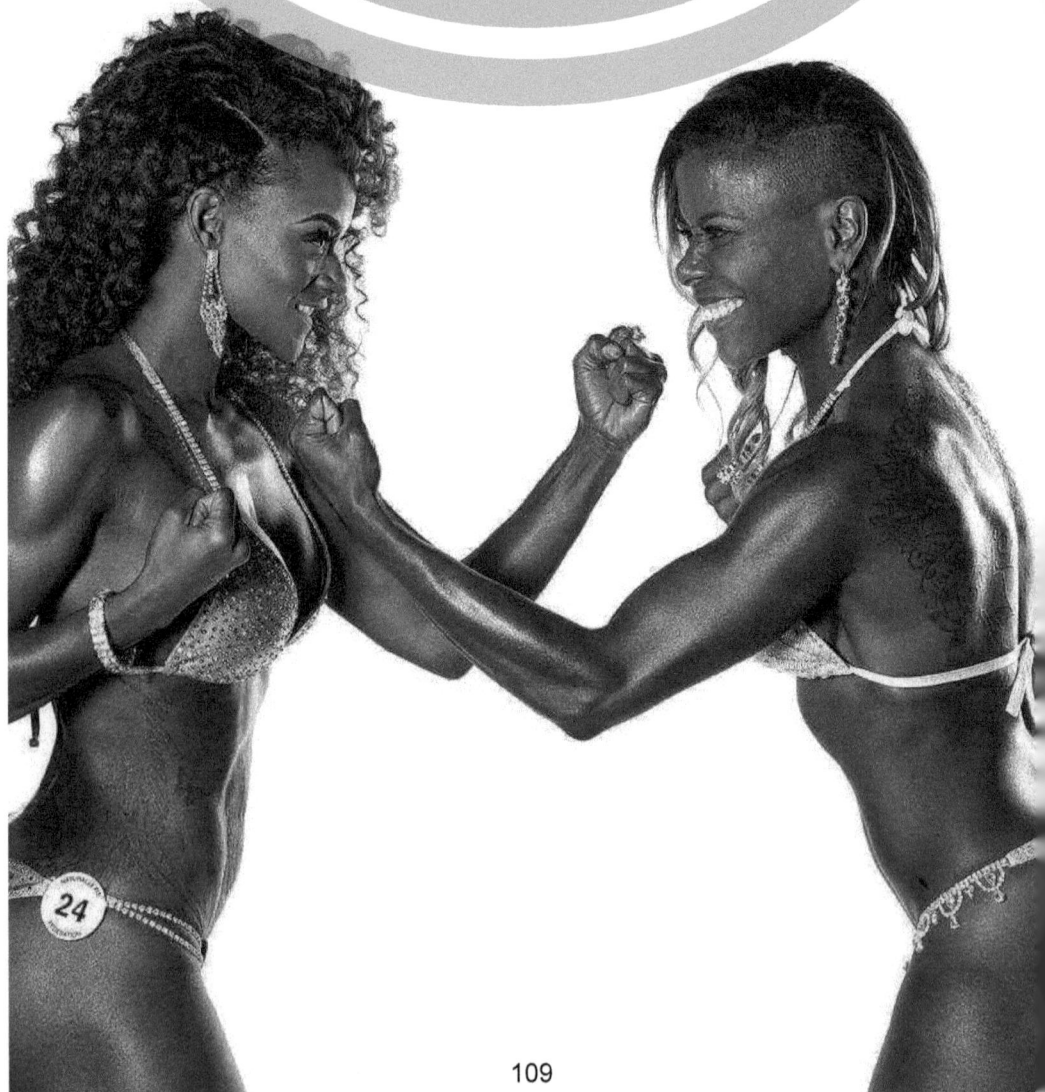

Super Moms

RULER OF YOUR OWN UNIVERSE

The hardest thing to accept is the fact that you hold the key to your own future. The seeds that you plant today determine the flowers that bloom tomorrow. So, plant good seeds and water them.

-JAMIE JAI

Helen Horton

Figure Pro Athlete

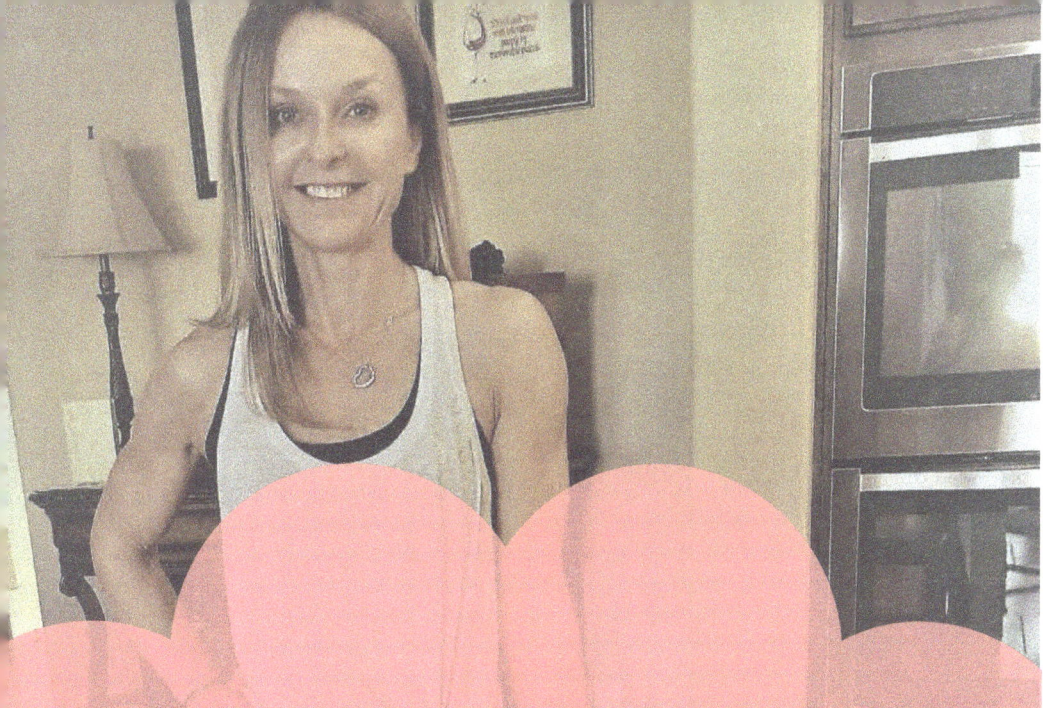

I am a figure competitor, mother of one, wife and nutritionist. I began bodybuilding in 2005. I had just had my son and was still carrying a bit of baby weight. After two years I experienced my first fitness competition. I have been competing ever since, except 18 months off due to a car accident in 2014. I write training plans and diets for many other competitors, and many wonder how I do it all. Planning, planning, planning! I make it a priority to organize and put family time and gym time on the calendar and commit to them. At times it is hard, but I gather inspiration from my husband, son, and my iron sisters. The challenges of being a working fit mom are keeping the balance between work, continuing professional development, and family time.

Thought it is hard it is not impossible because here I stand. The last three shows I competed in was The OCB Arizona Natural 2016; OCB Dessert City Classic 2014; OCB Yorton Cup 2013. I've been competing for ten years and going strong. The best is still to come.

I don't have a specific workout that I love. I workout based off a Daily Undulating Periodization workout program (DUP). DUP is a form of non-linear periodisation in which your training variables (volume and intensity) change on a per-session basis (source – Shredded by Science). Helps to create volume necessary for growth, without risk of over-training. Also keeps workouts fresh and interesting.

Favorite

Workout

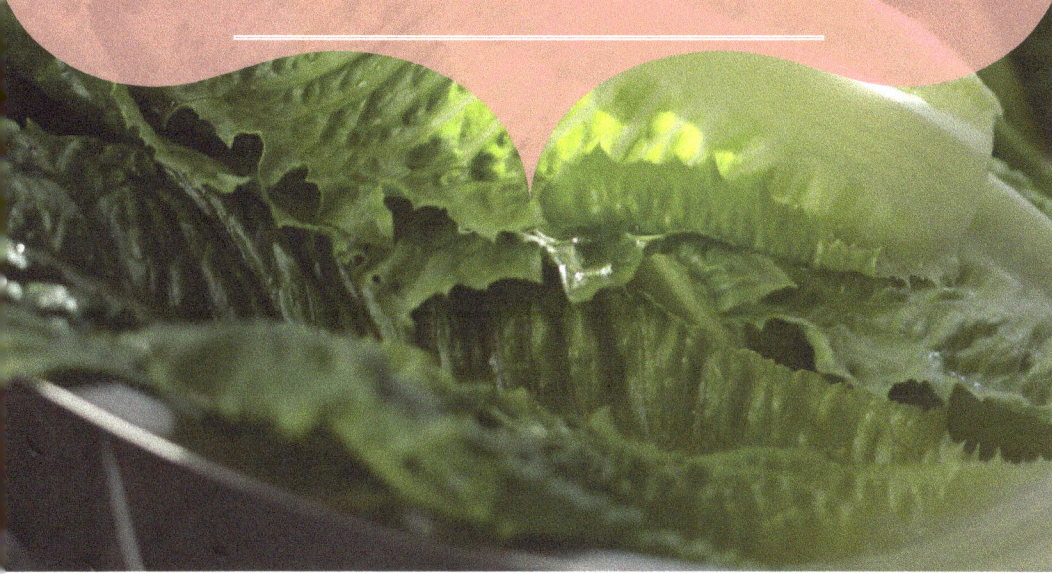

5 romaine leaves
3oz 99% lean ground turkey (cooked)
100g brown rice (measure cooked)
3oz avocado
2 tablespoons salsa

Protein 26g | Carbs 35g| Fats 15g

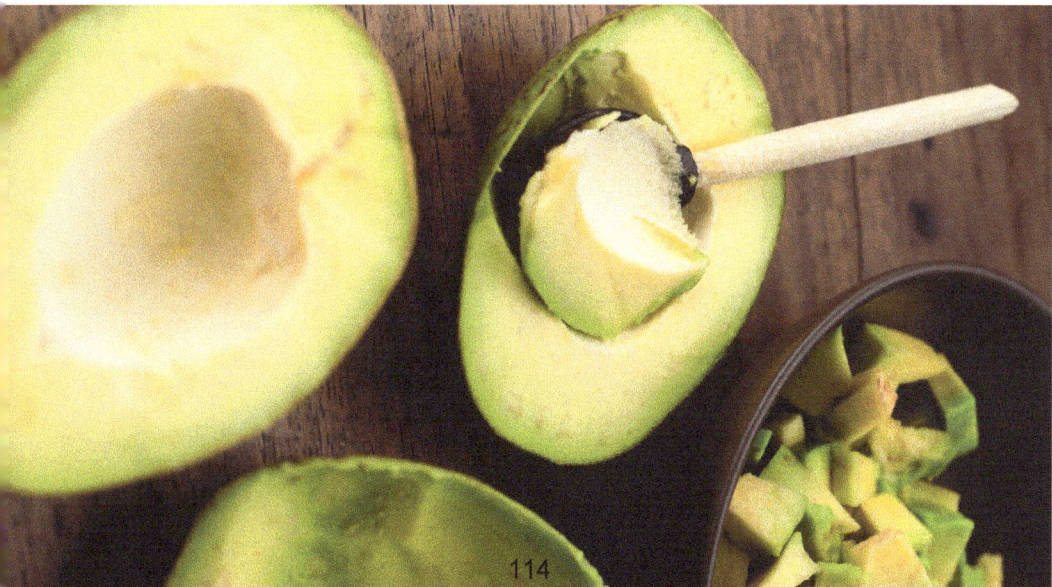

Muscle Tenderness

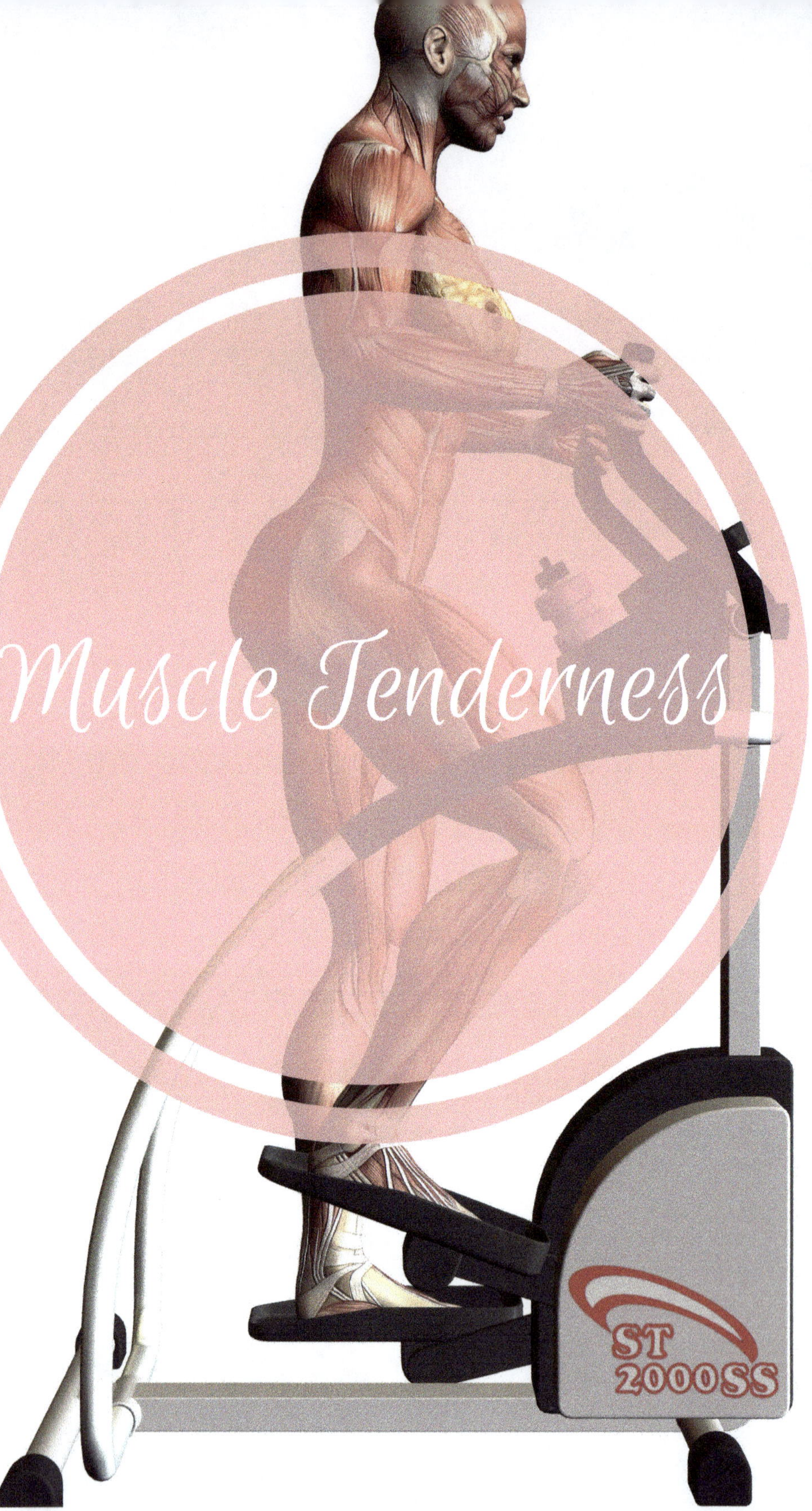

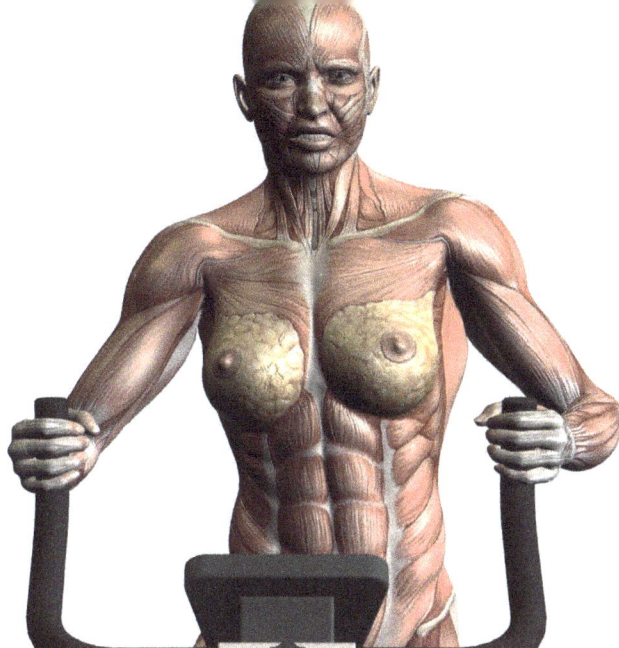

Myofascial Trigger Points

Muscle tenderness is normal when you have a good workout regimen. I like to call it "the painz of gains," but the pain you need to be concerned with are those that occur from an improper form or lifting too heavy of a weight.

We all are guilty of pushing ourselves a little further than we should when lifting and the majority of us fail to adequately stretch.

Stretching is one of the most important aspects of your workout. With stretching, you reduce the possibility for injury and allow full range of contraction. Failing to can lead to the development of muscle trigger points.

Myofascial trigger points are irritated areas in the fascia of skeletal muscle and are commonly called "knots."

When a muscle is under stretched it can lead to strains. The muscle then activates its protective action by constricting and tightening, which then leads to the muscle spasming as well as tenderness with movement or pressure.

The lack of relaxation leads to the development of these painful trigger points that then need to be treated by massaging, foam rolling, or trigger point injection of the affected area. Trigger Points can be broken down into two types. Active and latent.

Active trigger points are those that are new. They are the ones that you feel the day after injury and cause pain with movement. Latent trigger points are those that have been there for a while and are only tender when pressure is applied.

Stretching

So, how long should you stretch? The proper length of a stretch should be thirty seconds for each muscle. When you first start the stretch, you will feel the muscle fire off and spasm, but as you allow the thirty seconds to pass the muscle will relax.

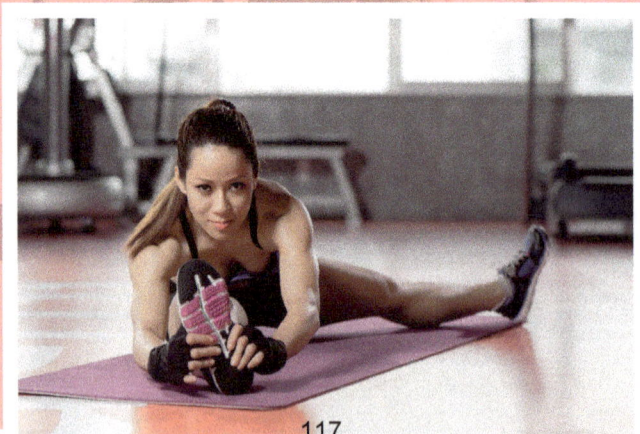

Let's be honest, stretching hurts for most, but for all, it helps maximize muscle growth. So, the best treatment after a strain is not to get back out there and lift again, but to give your muscle rest, gentle stretching, dry or moist heat and icing.

While dry heat can be more convenient, moist heat is known to penetrate deeper. It helps soothe the muscle and is a great benefit to stretching if applied before performing the stretch. Icing the muscle helps to reduce inflammation.

Inflammation is the biggest reason you feel the pain in the first place so icing with an anti-inflammatory can help improve pain.

When applying ice or heat, you don't apply the pack directly to the skin. Place a towel or thin material between skin and ice/heat pack and make sure you monitor skin for damage or decrease sensation. You should apply the pack for no more than 20 minutes twice a day.

When do you seek medical attention? You need to seek medical attention anytime you injure yourself especially if the injury results in mobility impairment, sensation change, weakness, swelling, color change and excruciating pain.

Treatment

The most common reasons for injury to these muscles is lack of proper stretching or small muscle group weakness.

For example, Plantar Fasciitis is a condition of inflammation of the fascia of the foot brought on by lack of stretching of the calf muscle. The calf muscle becomes tight, pulling on the Achilles tendon which inserts on the calcaneus bone in which the plantar fascia inserts also. Fascia is not as lax as tendon or muscle, and the pull on the Achilles leads to overstretching of the fascia leading to micro tears. Once plantar fasciitis is a problem, it is always a problem, so prevention is key.

Another commonly problematic area is the upper mid back. Your rhomboids are smaller muscles of the mid back and can be overpowered by the larger latissimus dorsi muscles that pull on the mid-back, which then strain the rhomboids. One great way to ensure you are working your rhomboids when rowing is to draw your shoulders back and maintain an erect posture during a workout.

Shoulder Rotator Cuff Muscles
Rhombiods
Upper & Lower Trapezuis
Plantar Fasciitis

Upper Crossed Syndrome (UCS) is a perfect example of unbalanced muscle tightness. Most trainers never really take the time to address this condition, but it is important to correct it to achieve maximal muscle growth, a full range of motion and flexibility when training.

What is UCS exactly? UCS is the tightness of the upper trapezius and levator scapula on the dorsal side with the tightness of the pectoralis major and minor. As time progresses and with lack of proper stretching those muscles get tighter leading to a forward curve in the shoulders which leads to a humpback appearance.

Your body likes to stay in homeostasis, and that includes your muscles.

The weakness of the deep cervical flexors ventrally crosses with weakness of the middle and lower trapezius.

This pattern of imbalance creates joint dysfunction, particularly at the atlanto-occipital joint, C4-C5 segment, cervicothoracic joint, glenohumeral joint, and T4-T5 segment.

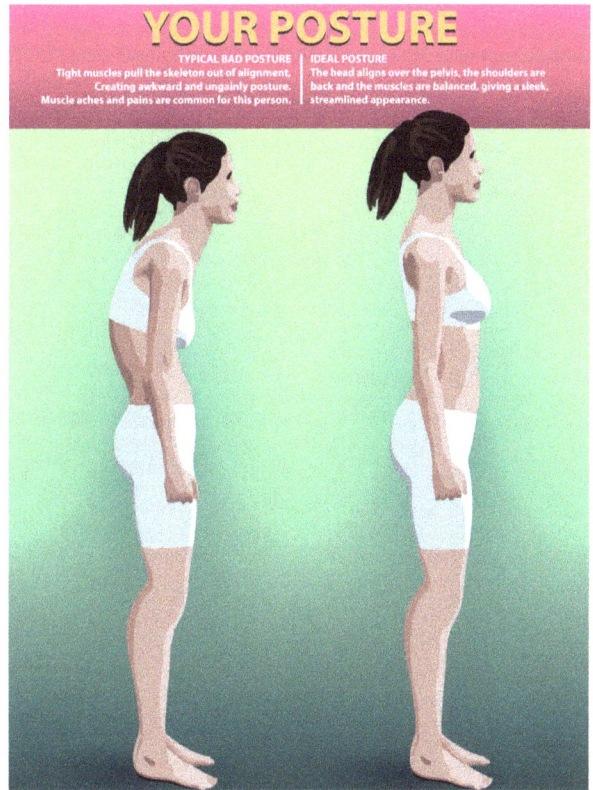

YOUR POSTURE

TYPICAL BAD POSTURE — Tight muscles pull the skeleton out of alignment. Creating awkward and ungainly posture. Muscle aches and pains are common for this person.

IDEAL POSTURE — The head aligns over the pelvis, the shoulders are back and the muscles are balanced, giving a sleek, streamlined appearance.

Therefore, it is important to work the small and large muscles of the body. The Rhomboids are smaller, and it's important to practice proper form to strengthen them as well stretching your shoulders and chest to prevent tightness.

Fixing this might take a little time. A trainer can encourage their client to go see a Physical Therapist or add these steps to training. First and foremost, working on good posture. Have the individual practice sitting or standing erect with shoulders relaxed and rolled back. Rolling the shoulders back should automatically elevate the chest. This step takes some getting used to. You are literally training your mind and muscle to hold a different posture.

After working on posture for a while, the next thing one should do is strengthening the smaller weaker muscles. Seated row and face pulls target these muscles. Because these muscles are smaller, you don't need heavy weight for them. Chose a lightweight and work your way up.

FIXING IT !

Lastly, stretch those chest and shoulder muscles. Remember an effective stretch will last 30 seconds.

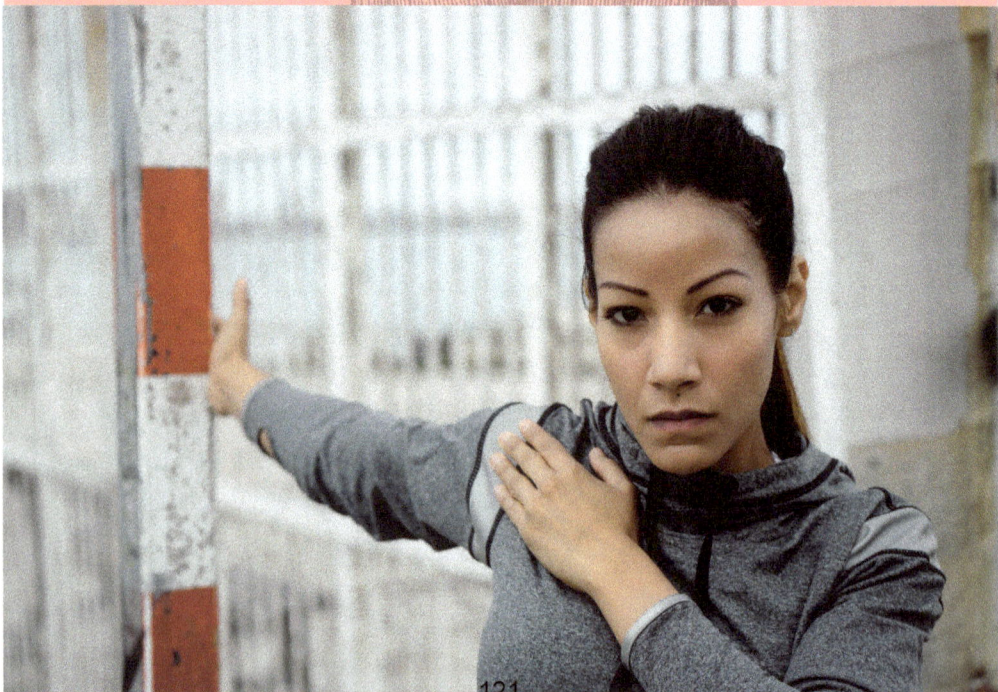

Failure to Treat Leads To

Headaches
Shoulder Pain
Back Pain
Neck Pain

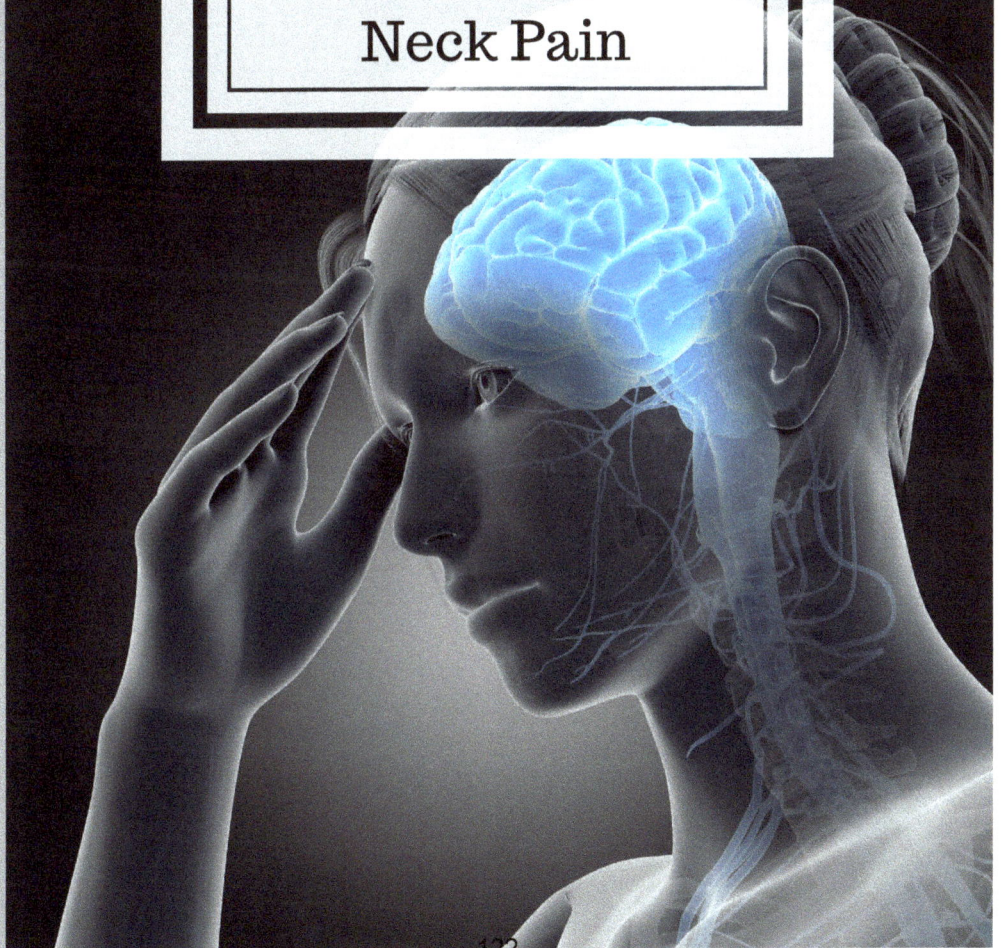

AB Work

WHY AREN'T MY ABS POPPING?

Abs are made in the kitchen. You can do a million crunches, but no amount of exercise out trains a bad diet.

When working abs, ask yourself whether you're trying to bulk or lean them. Structure the exercises to fit your goal. Lifting heavy weight with a low number of reps support bulking, so if you want a tiny waist, you might want to do lighter weights or body weighted exercises with a high number of reps. Remember for abs it's all about what you eat. Eat lean look lean!

Great Protein Options

Chicken breast
Turkey breast
Lean Red Meats
Tofu
fish
Egg whites
Nonfat cottage cheese
Protein Powder
Greek Yogurt
Black Beans
Red Beans
Lentils
Broccoli
Spinach

Training Them

Floor crunches
Reverse crunches
Twist crunches
Alternating heel touches
Windshield wipers
Leg raises
Flutter kicks
Bent knee leg raises
Planks
Weighted ab twist

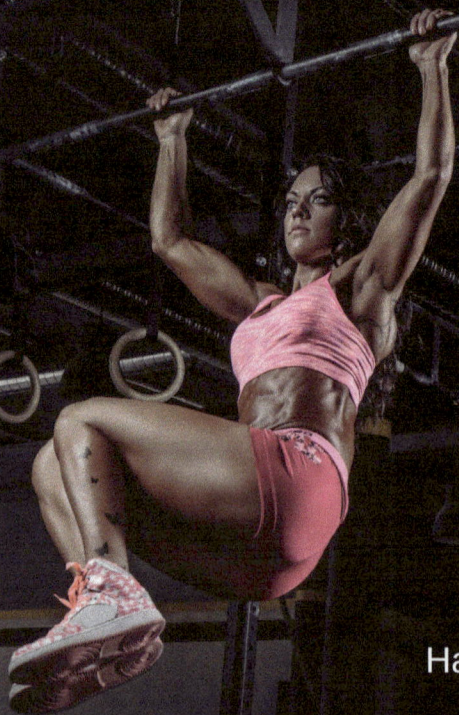

Hanging Knee Tucks

Healthy Fats

Chia seeds

Flax seeds

Avocado

Coconut oil

Pumpkin oil

Almond butter

Canola oil cooking spray

Natural peanut butter

Extra virgin olive oil

Raw nuts, cashews,
walnuts, almonds,
macadamia nuts, pumpkin
seeds

Body fat percentage plays an important role in those beach body abs. If you read my BMI & Body Fat Percentage chapter you will see they start to show when you're around 15-20% body fat. So, choose your fats wisely

Running For My Life

BE PREPARED

The infamous PT test! I can remember being terrified as that time of the year approached. I managed to always pass but had to start three months out preparing myself, but not anymore.

Taking care of your physical health on a daily basis can put you in place to never worry about whether you can pass or not. Now, I wonder whether or not I can get a perfect score.

It wasn't until I was a medic in a cop squadron that I took fitness seriously. One day I asked myself if I had to run for my life how far would I get? Then I asked myself if I had the strength and endurance to save others? At the time the answer was no. At that time, I knew that I couldn't run two miles without stopping and all the medic carries I learned would be a waste to try. I literally was a liability.

Watching the cops train embedded a deep respect for them in me and fostered the desire I needed to not be the weakest link in a battle. I started to value training alongside them learning to be vigilant and aware of my surroundings. The level of preparedness they had to have reminded me that I too could be outside the wire fighting right alongside them and the question of whether or not I could run to safety or carry a fallen was of huge importance to me.

I can now gauge how far someone is walking behind me and feel their presence before even seeing them. Then becoming fit wasn't about the look, it was about survival.

Now every day is about being prepared; whether it's being prepared to fight for your Country, pass a physical training test, run a marathon or compete in a bodybuilding competition.

Nothing you do ends in success if you don't train and practice for it. Don't be a sitting duck waiting to get sniped off. Prepare yourself for the known and unknown, because you never know what life will through your way.

Prepare

Plan

Execute

Succeed!!!

YOU ARE STRONGER THAN A TEMPORARY PITFALL

Never let your temporary deficiency decrease your dignity, allowing you to fall prey to those permanently undeserving of you

-JAMIE JAI

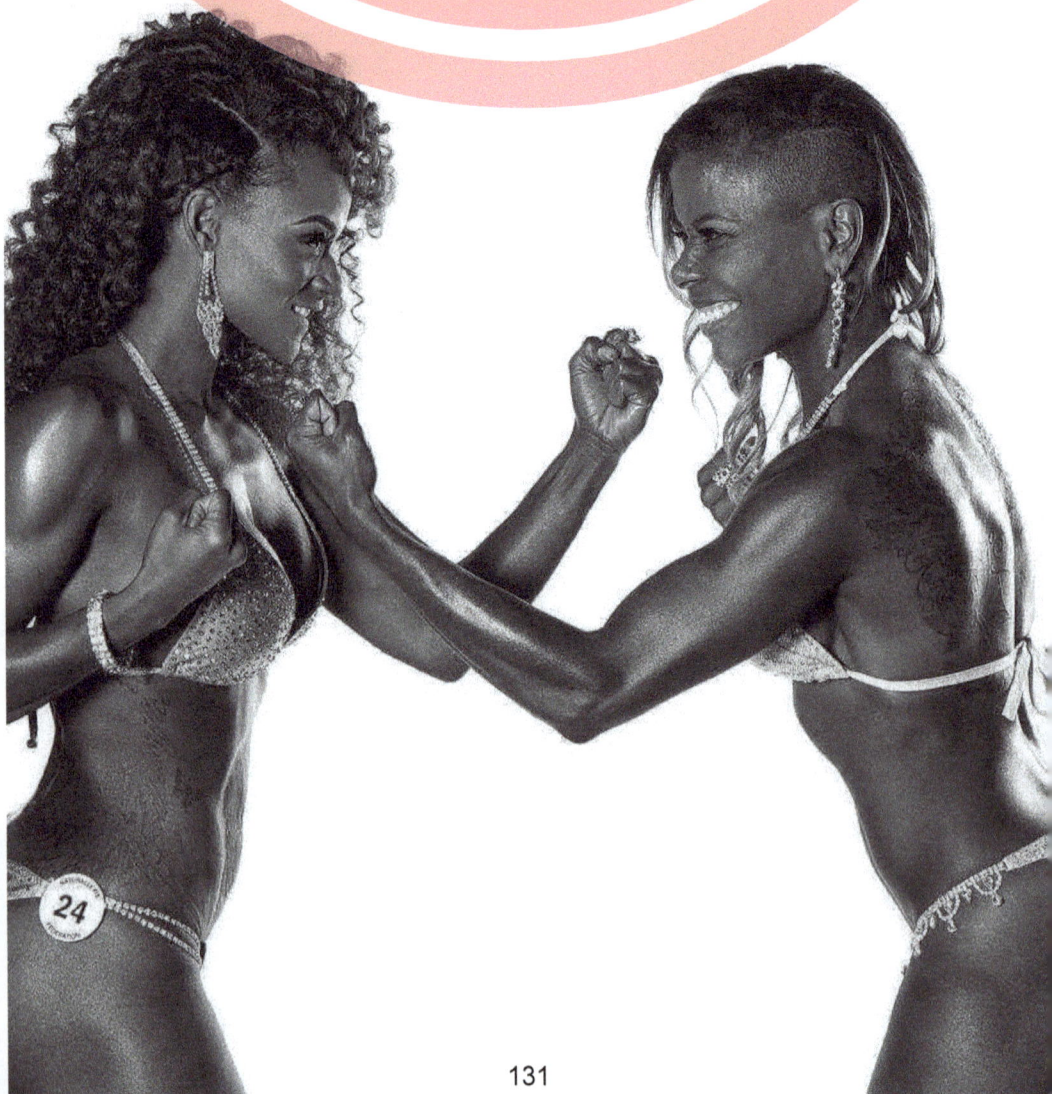

Super Moms

DETERMINATION

Would you live in a home or drive a vehicle that was half built? Of course not. We classify these types of things as unsafe, not sturdy or unreliable. So, why would you build an un-sturdy, unsafe and unreliable you?Build the best you, you can be. Strive for success and nothing less!

-JAMIE JAI

Sunni Ewing

Pro Bikini Athlete

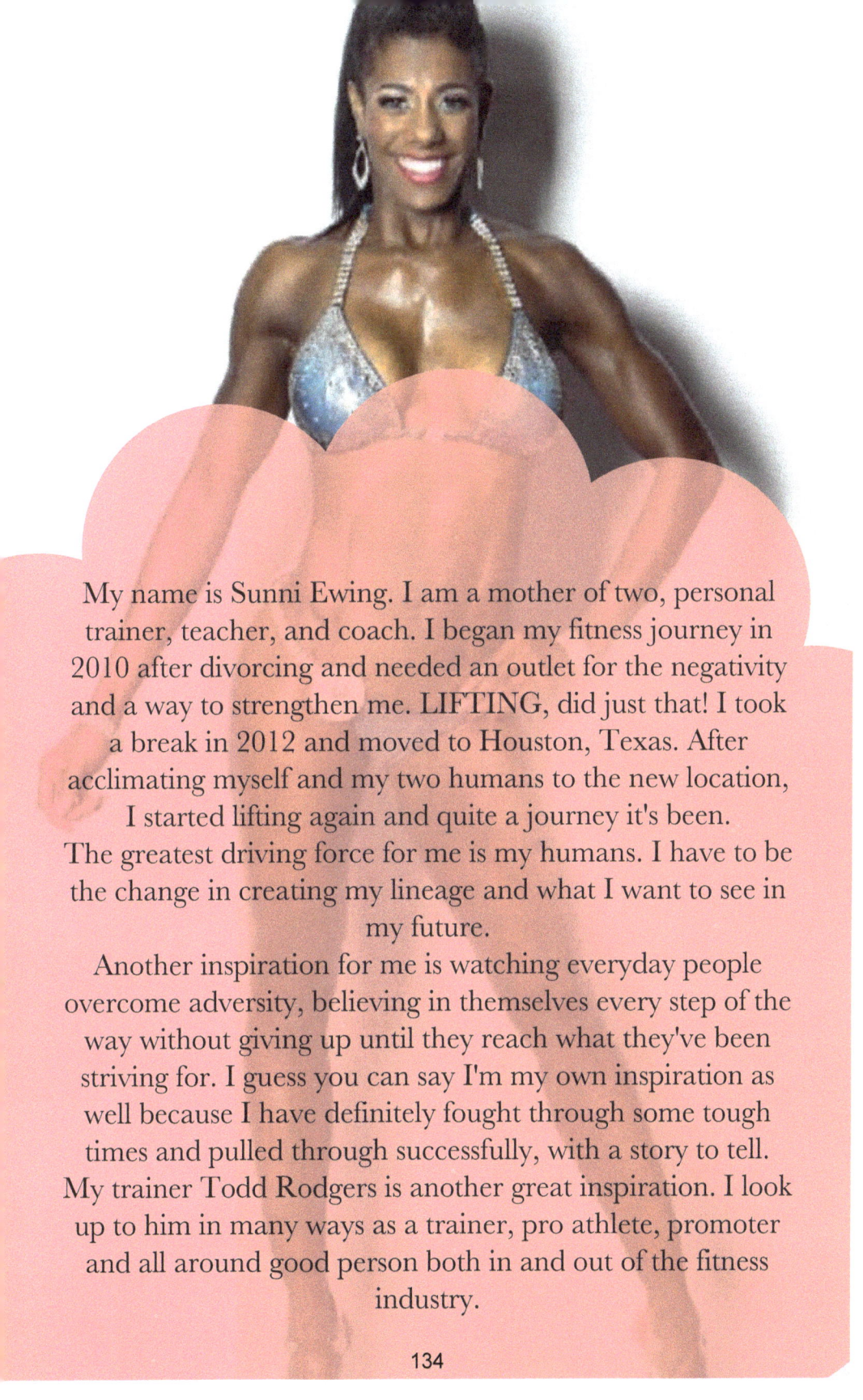

My name is Sunni Ewing. I am a mother of two, personal trainer, teacher, and coach. I began my fitness journey in 2010 after divorcing and needed an outlet for the negativity and a way to strengthen me. LIFTING, did just that! I took a break in 2012 and moved to Houston, Texas. After acclimating myself and my two humans to the new location, I started lifting again and quite a journey it's been.

The greatest driving force for me is my humans. I have to be the change in creating my lineage and what I want to see in my future.

Another inspiration for me is watching everyday people overcome adversity, believing in themselves every step of the way without giving up until they reach what they've been striving for. I guess you can say I'm my own inspiration as well because I have definitely fought through some tough times and pulled through successfully, with a story to tell. My trainer Todd Rodgers is another great inspiration. I look up to him in many ways as a trainer, pro athlete, promoter and all around good person both in and out of the fitness industry.

One of the biggest challenges I've faced being a fit mom is not so much the fitness and mothering, but more the pressure to model correct behavior for my humans.

I have to remember that my humans are watching me in all areas of my life and I must see all goals through. When I fall, it is vital that they see me get back up. My children see me as the first example of how to deal with life's obstacles.

At times I might feel tired and stressed, but balance is key. I also believe that you have to embrace the challenges in life and know that they shape you into who you are meant to be. The main objective is not to break, but to keep moving forward.

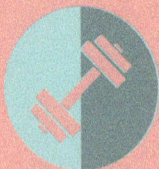

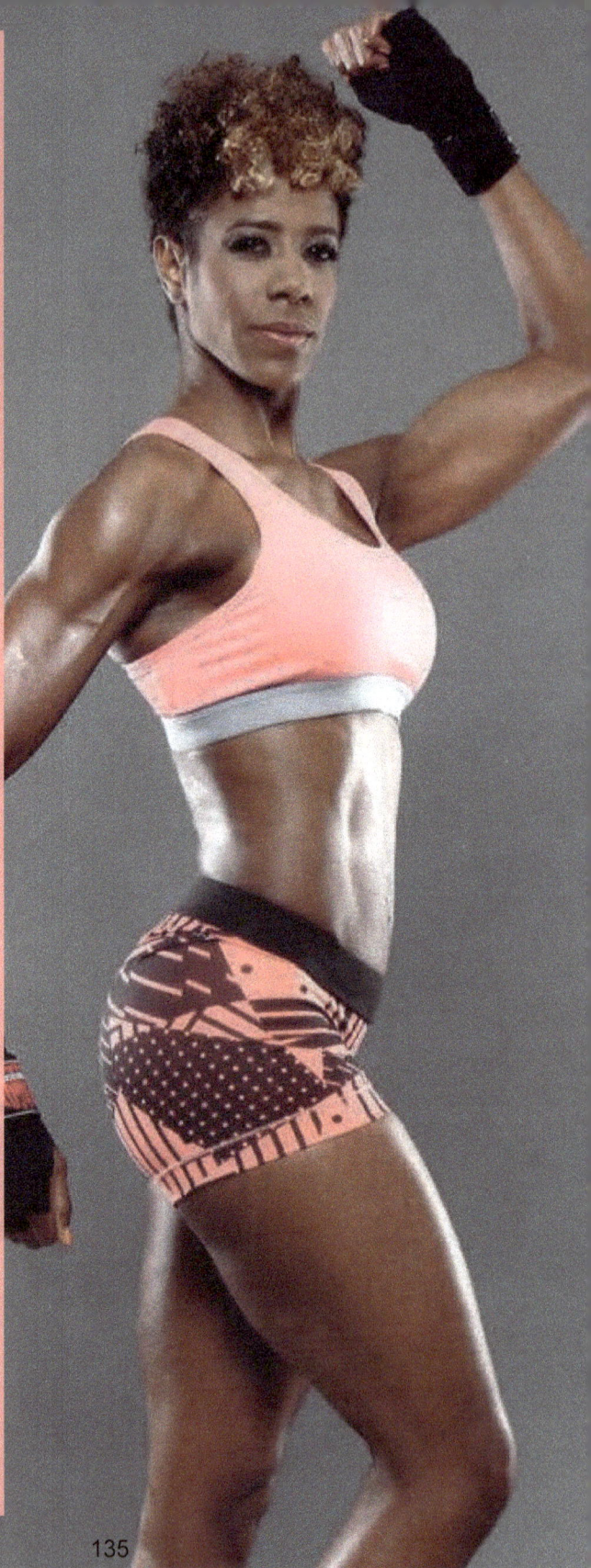

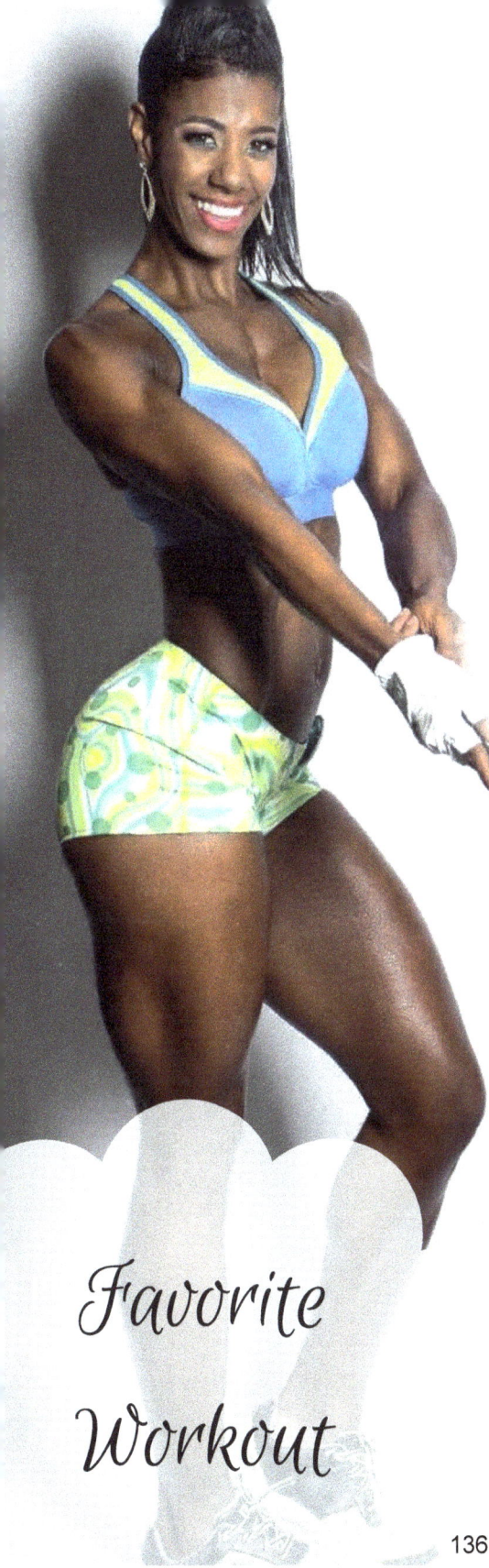

My favorite workout would have to be the Hip Belt Weighted Squats. It works the Gluteus muscles very well and gives them that nice round appearance.

I will do eight heavy sets at eight to twelve reps. All you need is a hip belt, the heavy weight of choice and place feet on an elevated surface (i.e., step-ups, or low boxes) then bend down as if you were doing a squat and raise yourself back up squeezing those glutes as you come back up.

Favorite

Workout

FAVORITE MEAL

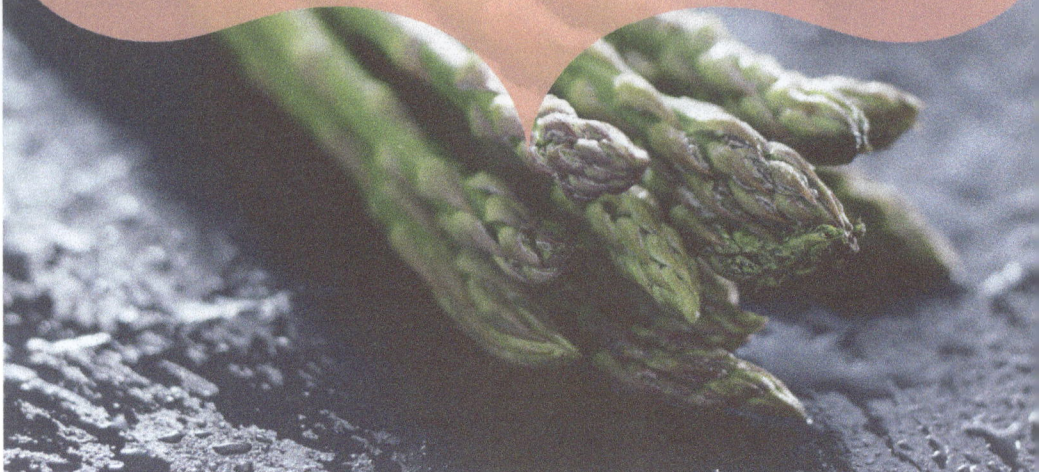

4.5oz Chilean Sea Bass
6 Spears of Asparagus
1 Cup of Jasmine Rice
1/4 Small Avocado

Protein 31.9g | Carbs 56.4g| Fats 9.3g

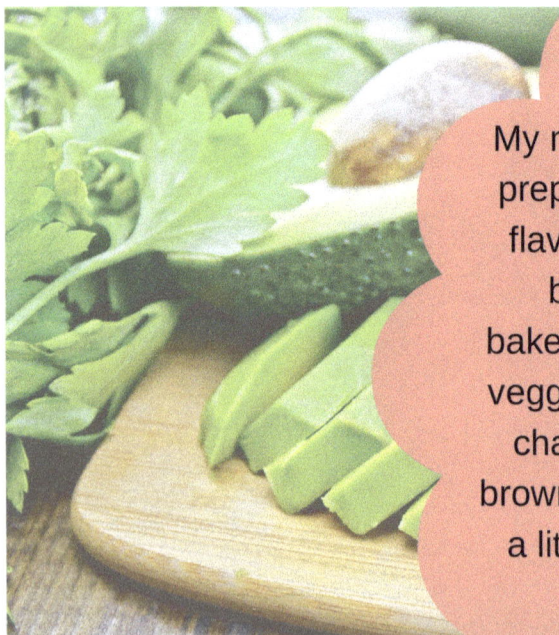

My meal Plan is pretty fulfilling on prep. I like to snack on chocolate flavored rice cakes with almond butter. My favorite meal is baked chilean sea bass and green veggies with brown rice. At times I change it up by substituting my brown rice with sweet potatoes and a little Avocado seals the meal!

KNOW YOUR OWN STRENGTH

Never let your strength be determined by your number of failures, but by the number of times you got up when you fell

-JAMIE JAI

The Bikini

Toxic Angel Bikinis

The bikini can make or break you. Of course, you feel like the more bling, the better, but too much bling can actually be distracting. You want your physique to stand out more than your suit. Yes, the overall appearance is of value and beauty is admired, but it is the hard work put in from hitting the gym and sticking to your diet that will get you the win.

What if you don't have that many funds, but you still want a decent quality suit? Well get crafty and stone the suit yourself. If you bought a basic suit a few months out, you would have enough time to add stones to it.

Some might say they aren't crafty, but when you have to choose between $100 and $600 you will be, or you don't want to save money.

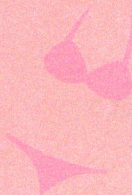

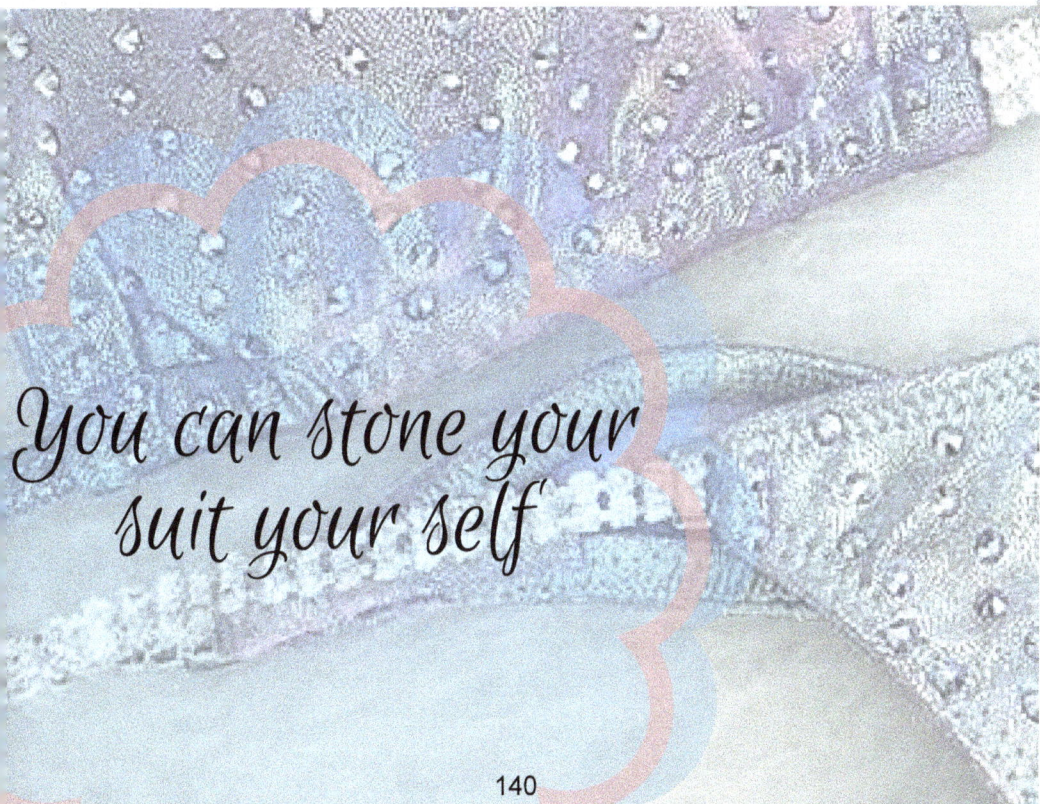

You can stone your suit your self

You Don't Need A New One Each Show!

Buying suits can be addicting. It's like buying a new purse or getting your nails done. Some competitors even use it as a way to keep them motivated for their show, but the truth is you don't need a new suit for every show.

As long as your suit compliments your skin tone and still looks nice you should use it. You could actually choose a well-made basic suit whose color perfectly matches your skin tone and add stones each show that you do. Depending on how you stone it you can create a new look with the same suit.

The most important thing is purchasing a suit that will hold up against the tan. For example, a white suit is absolutely stunning on some skin tones, but it is so easily damaged by the tan. Therefore, if you are trying to keep cost low to compete, a white suit in regard to longevity might not be the suit for you.

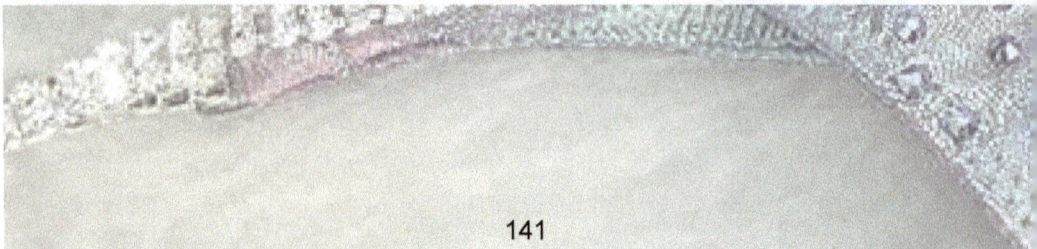

I am a believer in the phrase quality over quantity. The worst thing you can do is have a bunch of poor quality shoes, clothes, or suits. I say this because they will wear out fast and you will need to replace them often leading you to spend more money in the long run.

So, I always recommend saving your money to have a high-quality suit made. It will also reduce the chance of suit malfunction. Some malfunctions aren't a quick fix, and I have never been to a show where the suit maker was there to fix anything. So, make sure you get a quality suit and test it out before show day.

If you have to get a cheap suit, get it because it's your back up suit and trust me, a judge can tell when a suit is high quality or not.

Quality Over Quantity

Your Show Day Checklist

Everyone's list varies, but it's important to have down the basics. Make sure you know who is doing your makeup/tan and when. If you are doing them, then do test runs weeks out so that things flow easier for the show and you know how much time it will take you to do these things

- Competition Suits
- Clear Heels
- Earrings
- Bracelet
- Robe
- Loose Fitting Clothing
- Flip Flops
- Federation Card
- Make-up Kit & Hair
- After Show outfit for celebration
- Bikini Bite
- Meals
- Rice Cakes & Almond Butter, Rice Crispy Treats or what ever you will use to carb up with and for pump back stage.
- Water & a small bottle of Pedialyte or Gatorade to replenish electrolytes after show
- Phone Charger
- Sewing Kit

WHAT FEDERATION IS RIGHT FOR ME?

You Get to Decide!

When thinking about what federation you want to compete in, you need to figure out which category you want to be in. Then after looking at your body habitus and choosing the category that best fits your physique look at a few pro athletes from that federation. It is important for you to understand what that federation is looking for. This will save you a lot of time and as well as money.

Now, you need to sit down and ask yourself if you want to be a natural athlete or would you be willing to take supplements containing hormones for additional growth. Natural organizations lie detector test as well as perform a urinalysis to ensure that their athletes have not used any banned substances.

NATURAL FEDERATIONS

ABA/INBA/PNBA
Presents Natural Olympia

ABFF
Alaska Bodybuilding, Fitness
and Figure

ANBF
American Natural
Bodybuilding Federation

BNBF
British Natural Bodybuilding
Federation

DFAC
Drug Free Athletes Coalition

FAME World Tour
Amateur and Pro Physique
competitions worldwide that
lead into the World
Championships

Fitness Universe™ Celebrating
25th Anniversary Season

IDFA
International Drug Free
Athletics

IPE
International Pro Elite

IPL
International Physique League

INBA Canada
International Natural
Bodybuilding Association of
Canada

IFBB Pro League
International Federation of
Body Building and Fitness

Model World Tour

IFBB Physique America

Musclemania®
Celebrating 25th Anniversary
Season

NANBF
North American Natural
Bodybuilding Federation NMA
Natural Muscle Association

NBFI
Federazione Natural
Bodybuilding and Fitness Italy

NFF
Naturally Fit Federation

NGA
National Gym Association

NIFMA
Northern Ireland Fitness Model
Association

NPA – US
National Physique Association
(United States)

NPA – UK
National Physique Association
(United Kingdom)

NPAA
Natural Physique and Athletics
Association (Canada)
NPC
National Physique Commitee

NASF
North American Sports
Federation
Iron Sports Division is a non- profit
educational, officiating and
program coordinating body for
amateur adults and youth athletes
participating in bodybuilding,
power lifting and Olympic
weightlifting.
OCB
Organization of Competitive
Bodybuilders

USBF
United States Bodybuilding
Federation

WBFMA
World Beauty Fitness Model
Association

WNBF
World Natural Bodybuilding
Federation

WPA
World Physique Alliance

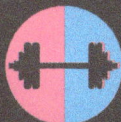

Meal Prepping

MAGNIFY THE POSITIVE

You can't control what comes into
your life, but you decide what you
magnify

-JAMIE JAI

Meal Prep Tips

1. Keep your prep simple when starting out, make a list and never shop while hungry.
2. Break up your prep in two days. You can prep on a Sunday and then use Wednesday as a day to do a small prep to replenish your meals or prep for the last part of the week.

3. Know your favorite meals and comfort foods. Research ahead of time for healthier substitutes. You don't exactly have to give up the foods you love, but making them with fewer ingredients on your own or replacing them with something similar and healthier will reduce the feeling of missing out on them.

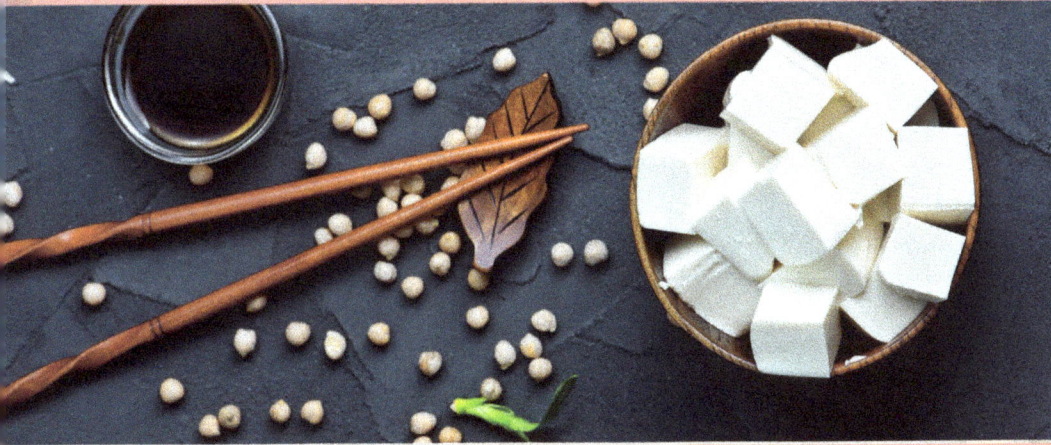

4. Portion control is everything! Even if you don't use macros to manage weight, it is still a good idea to buy a food scale and weigh your foods so you can become familiar with the right portion size for you. This reduces the chance of overeating when you are out because you will become familiar with eye balling how much you can eat.

Tofu is a great source of protein

5. If you are a macro tracker, which I am, there are a variety of apps available for macro tracking. Get one!

Slow Cooker Meals Are A Life saver When It Comes to Prep

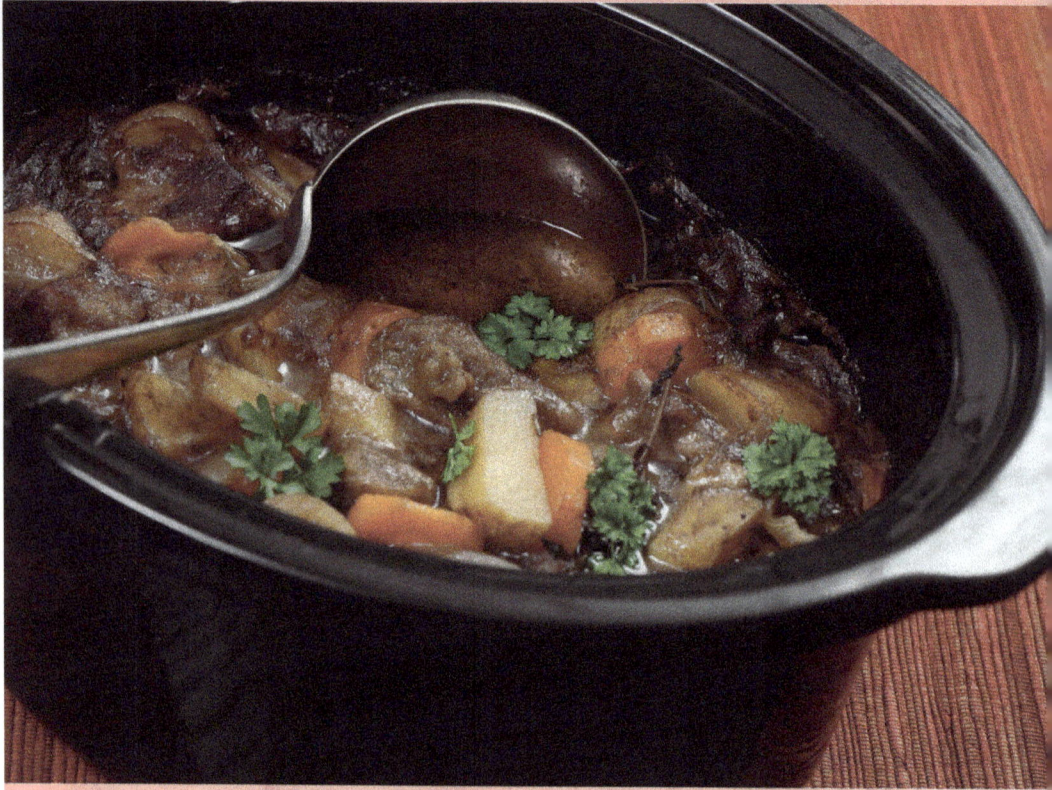

6. Find shortcuts to help make cooking easier. Frozen veggies are a great option for this and are way better than canned veggies.

7. Reduce the amount of food temptation you have in the home. Instead of getting those double stuffed Oreos, get the thin ones and limit how many you can have a day, or better yet, have the willpower not buy them at all. I am a huge snacker myself, so I have to have at least one snack alternative to turn to.

8. Ensure you prepare your water or at least have a plan in place for water intake.

9. SCHEDULE YOUR EARNED MEALS! Many refer to these meals as cheat meals, but technically it's not cheating if you have put in the work to indulge. Calling it a cheat meal is associating it with something bad, and it isn't. It's a meal you have scheduled as a reward for all your hard work.

10. Don't be hard on yourself. Eating habits are more than just a change involving actions. It involves physical, mental and emotional change. It is going to take a while for your mind and body to act in unison for the goals you have set for yourself.

When you meal prep you're more likely to eat what you have made when you're hungry rather than to just go grab something from somewhere that may or may not be healthy.

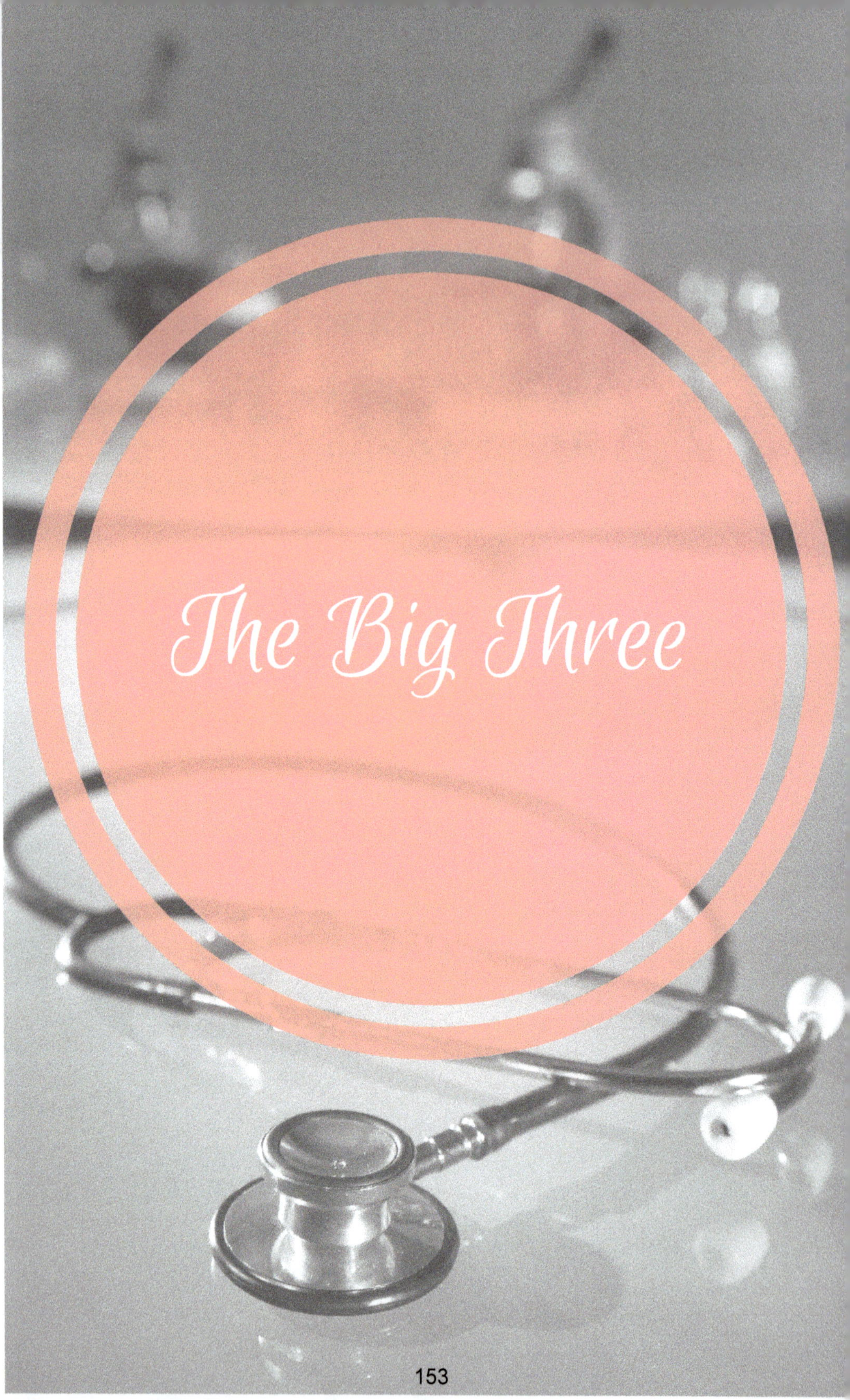

The Big Three

NEVER GIVE UP

You've started the process and gotten over the initial fear of entering the unknown. Things are still not quite clear, but you have built up the drive to put in the work to accomplish your goals. All you must do now is remain true to yourself and see the journey to the end. You have to dig deep and persist until something great happens. It's an uphill battle some days, but you have to yell, "I will never give up." Whether you reach the moon or the stars, you've made it somewhere, and that is way better than surrendering to self-doubt. All you need to do now is believe in yourself!

-JAMIE JAI

High Cholesterol

High Blood Pressure

Diabetes

Earlier in this book we discussed high blood pressure, diabetes and high cholesterol. I like to call these diseases the "Big Three". During my time practicing medicine I realized that these three diseases follow each other. Meaning, if you don't get one under control than your risk of developing the other two is higher.

A large amount of patients with the Big Three have a BMI or fat percentage over thirty. Notice I used the term BMI and not obese. Just because you appear to be what society views as "skinny" doesn't mean that you are internally healthy.

It is a misconception that if you are "skinny" you are not at risk for developing these diseases. Remember, It is about the ratio of fat to muscle. So yes, one's appearance can be slim, but if your body fat is high then you are still at risk for developing high blood pressure, diabetes and high cholesterol. Regardless of whether or not you look slim or look obese it's very important to understand how the Big Three decreases your quality of life and can quickly lead you to death's door.

Atherosclerotic Cardiovascular Disease (ASCVD)
ASCVD is most often caused by uncontrolled high blood pressure and high cholesterol. This disease puts patients at risk of heart attack. The blood vessels of the heart get clogged with fatty deposits when cholesterol is high.

The fatty deposits can embed in the tears caused by high blood pressure and set off a hormonal cascade that leads to the development of a blood clot. This blood clot can then break free and roam through vessels until it lodges in the smaller vessels of the heart or even the brain. Blood flow is decreased and the tissue around the clot starves for oxygen then dies.

ASCVD is just one of many examples of what the Big Three can lead to. Uncontrolled high blood pressure alone causes damage to the liver as well as kidneys. When accompanied by diabetes liver and kidney failure occurs much quicker.

As I stated before, it's not all about how you look on the outside and sometimes it's not even bout how you feel. These diseases can silently destroy your organs, limbs and lead to vision loss.

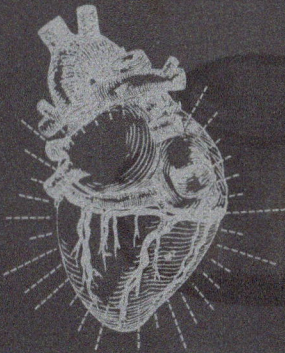

What The Big Three Lead To

Today the battle with obesity and excess weight is high. Older adults use to make up the majority of the patient population with health issues, but now there is a growing concern in those as young as eleven years old.

Many people have busy lives and resort to the quickest, which is not always the healthiest, option for food. We feed these foods to our children and to be quite honest don't pay attention to the portion size.

One day I took a fast food place's children's meal and looked at the macro break down as well as the calories. What I realized is that I was feeding my children half of their recommended daily caloric intake; not to mention the meal was 35% fat.

At this moment I learned it's not just about what I put in my body, but also my children's. I was feeding my kids something that would lead them to have childhood obesity and lacked the nutrients needed for their growth. Instead of feeding them to death I made the choice to feed them to life.

Eat Your Self To Life

WHAT IS YOUR LEGACY?

A spirit is nothing more than an energy marking a place in a space of time. When all is said and done what type of energy will you leave behind

-JAMIE JAI

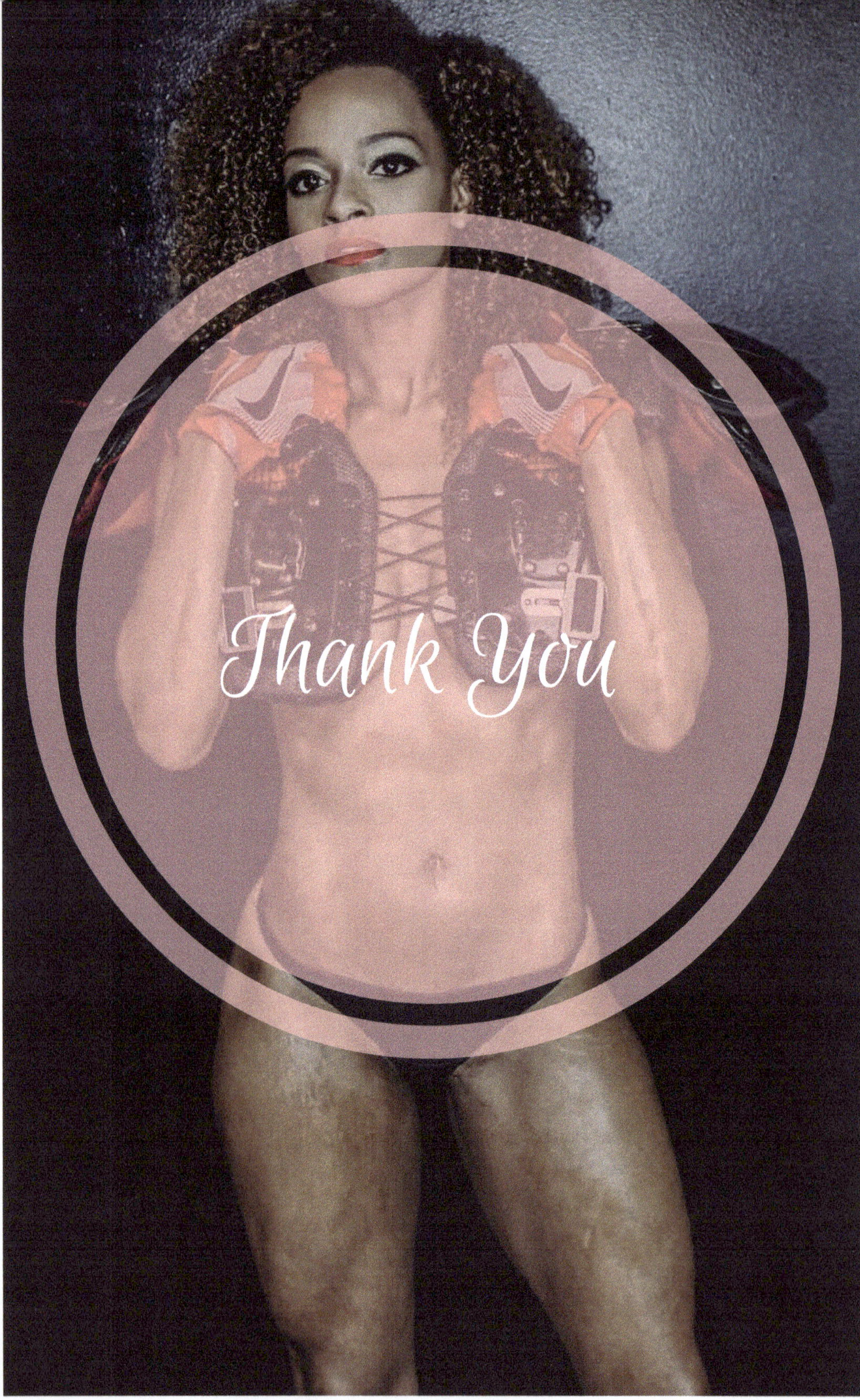

Thank You

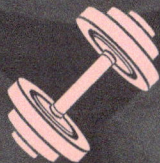

www.ingramcontent.com/pod-product-compliance
Lightning Source LLC
Chambersburg PA
CBHW042247040426
42334CB00044B/3060